疟疾
能在地球上
消失吗？

Can We Get Rid of
Malaria on Earth?

主　编　周晓农
副主编　肖　宁　张　仪

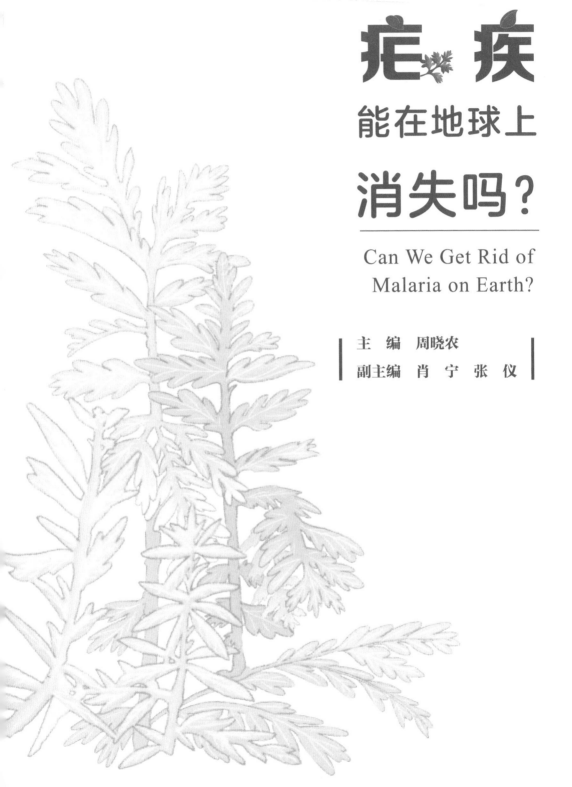

Editorial Committee

编委会

主 编

周晓农　中国疾病预防控制中心寄生虫病预防控制所（国家热带病研究中心）

副主编

肖　宁　中国疾病预防控制中心寄生虫病预防控制所（国家热带病研究中心）
张　仪　中国疾病预防控制中心寄生虫病预防控制所（国家热带病研究中心）

审　阅（按姓氏拼音排序）

蔡　黎　上海市疾病预防控制中心
郭　岩　北京大学公共卫生学院
黎　浩　武汉大学公共卫生学院
夏志贵　中国疾病预防控制中心寄生虫病预防控制所（国家热带病研究中心）
姚立农　浙江省疾病预防控制中心
周水森　中国疾病预防控制中心寄生虫病预防控制所（国家热带病研究中心）

编　者（按姓氏拼音排序）

陈伟奇　河南省疾病预防控制中心
邓　艳　河南省疾病预防控制中心
方　圆　中国疾病预防控制中心寄生虫病预防控制所（国家热带病研究中心）
李红梅　中国疾病预防控制中心寄生虫病预防控制所（国家热带病研究中心）
李卫东　安徽省疾病预防控制中心
李元元　中国疾病预防控制中心寄生虫病预防控制所（国家热带病研究中心）
李中秋　中国疾病预防控制中心寄生虫病预防控制所（国家热带病研究中心）
林康明　广西壮族自治区疾病预防控制中心
刘　琴　中国疾病预防控制中心寄生虫病预防控制所（国家热带病研究中心）
刘　颖　河南省疾病预防控制中心
罗　飞　重庆市疾病预防控制中心
吕　山　中国疾病预防控制中心寄生虫病预防控制所（国家热带病研究中心）
王多全　中国疾病预防控制中心寄生虫病预防控制所（国家热带病研究中心）
王新宇　复旦大学附属华山医院
许建卫　云南省寄生虫病防治所
杨丽敏　中国疾病预防控制中心寄生虫病预防控制所（国家热带病研究中心）
张红卫　河南省疾病预防控制中心
周瑞敏　河南省疾病预防控制中心

Editorial Committee

编委会

翻 译（按姓氏拼音排序）

丁 玮　中国疾病预防控制中心寄生虫病预防控制所（国家热带病研究中心）

科库维·卡森涅　上海交通大学医学院－国家热带病研究中心全球健康学院

李红梅　中国疾病预防控制中心寄生虫病预防控制所（国家热带病研究中心）

陆申宁　中国疾病预防控制中心寄生虫病预防控制所（国家热带病研究中心）

马雪娇　中国疾病预防控制中心寄生虫病预防控制所（国家热带病研究中心）

插 画

张子扬　上海交通大学设计学院

鸣 谢：上海市科学技术协会，中国疾病预防控制中心

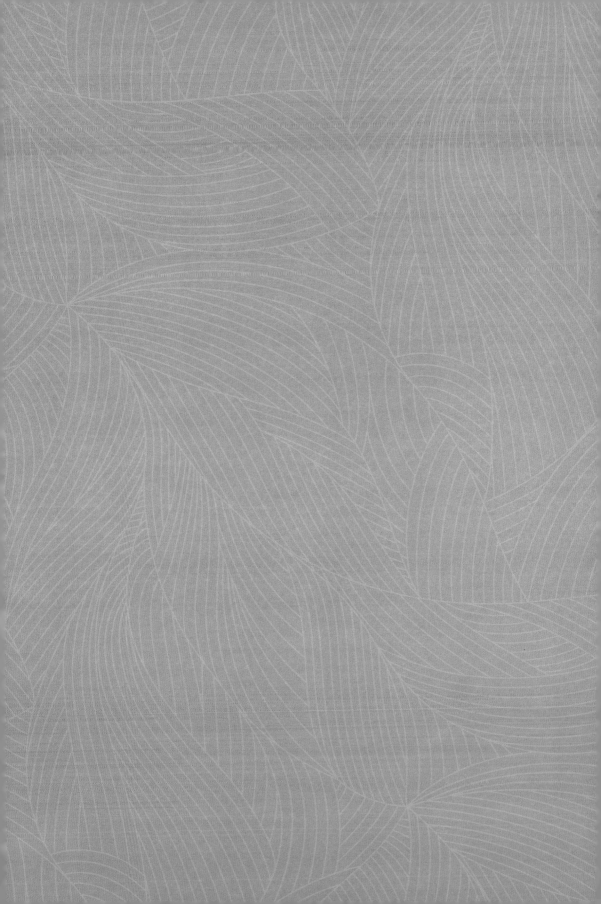

Preface

Malaria is an ancient infectious disease transmitted by mosquitoes, which has caused infinite detriment to human beings. It is recorded that malaria has existed on the earth for over 30 million years, and it killed totally 100 million people from 1910s to 1950s alone. Both Alexander the Great, who swept across Europe, Asia and Africa, and Dante, a well-known scholar who wrote *The Divine Comedy*, not to mention those nameless civilians, all lost their lives due to malaria. Malaria even played a crucial role in the outcome of historical wars, resulting in the change of the destiny of a country. Malaria has posed enormous challenges to human beings. Today, many parts of the world are still under the threats of malaria. In China, malaria had been prevalent for at least 3,000 years, and it was rather harmful, causing a large number of deaths. Before 1949, there were 30 million cases of malaria every year. In June 2021, the World Health Organization (WHO) announced that malaria had been eliminated in China. After the establishment of the People's Republic of China, thanks to more than 70 years of hard work by several generations, the number of people suffering from malaria in China has dropped from 30 million cases per year to zero cases at present, achieving the great feat of malaria-free in China.

However, can malaria be eradicated from the earth? This is not only a long-cherished wish of mankind, but a scientific problem. To this end, residents in endemic regions all over the world as well as international professional organizations have a hope that the innovative science and technology advancements such as the "anti-malaria miracle medicine" artemisinin and "1-3-7" work norm in the phase of eliminating malaria in China, and the practical prevention and control experience such as "barefoot doctors" and "patriotic health campaign" can be shared with those countries where malaria is still prevalent, so as to prevent people in these countries from suffering from malaria.

For this purpose, we have presented China's precious experience accumulated over these years to more countries and people in the form of popularization of science, and by means of excellent pictures and accompanying essays, demonstrated how people in China prevented and controlled malaria, how medical

前　言

疟疾是一种非常古老的、经蚊虫传播的传染病，对人类造成了巨大危害。据记载，疟疾已经在地球上存在了 3 000 多万年，仅 20 世纪 10 年代至 50 年代，疟疾就夺去了 1 亿人的生命。无论是横扫欧亚非的亚历山大大帝，还是创作出《神曲》的著名学者但丁，更不用说那些寂寂无闻的平民百姓，都因疟疾而失去生命。疟疾甚至影响了历史上战争的结局，进而改变了国家的命运。疟疾给人类带来了巨大挑战，如今全球仍有很多地区处于疟疾的威胁之中。在中国，疟疾至少流行了 3 000 年，并且危害深重，造成大量人群死亡。1949 年以前每年疟疾患者达 3 000 万。2021 年 6 月，世界卫生组织宣布中国消除了疟疾。中华人民共和国成立后，经过几代人 70 多年的艰苦努力，中国患疟疾的人数从每年 3 000 万降至如今的 0，实现了消除疟疾这一伟大壮举。

但是，疟疾能否从地球上彻底消失？这既是人类的一个夙愿，也是一个科学问题。为此，世界各地疟疾流行区居民及国际专业机构均有一个希望，将中国消除疟疾历程中创新的"抗疟神药：青蒿素"、"1-3-7"工作规范等技术产品和"赤脚医生""爱国卫生运动"等实用的防控经验分享给目前还在流行疟疾的国家，使这些国家的民众免受疟疾的伤害。

为此，我们以科普的形式，将中国多年积累的宝贵经验分享给更多的国家和民众，以图文并茂的形式，展现中国民众如何预防控制疟疾、医疗卫生机构如何应对疟疾流行、当地政府如何协调管理各项疟疾防控工作，以及中国公共卫生专家如何响应"一带一路"倡议，为人类卫生健康共同体作出贡献。

and health facilities response to malaria endemic, how local governments managed all sorts of malaria prevention and control programmes in coordination, and how Chinese public health experts responded to the Belt and Road Initiative in China-Africa cooperation and made contributions to a global community of health for all.

This scientific education book is composed of five parts and 36 sections, with over 100 illustrations and 12 case studies. It is designed to benefit people in different countries on the prevention and control of malaria, allow professionals in malaria-endemic countries to learn the practices of eliminating malaria in China and share china's experience in malaria control with malaria endemic countries.

本科普书分 5 个部分 36 节，共有插图百余幅，案例分析 12 个，力求使不同国家的民众了解疟疾防控知识，让疟疾流行国家的专业人员学习到中国消除疟疾的做法，与疟疾流行国家分享中国治理疟疾的经验。

CONTENTS

4. Prevention and Control in Endemic Regions

4. 疫情防控

5. 治　疗

5. Treatment

011

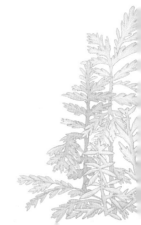

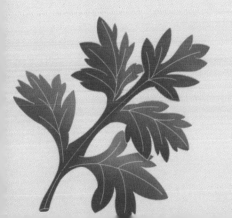

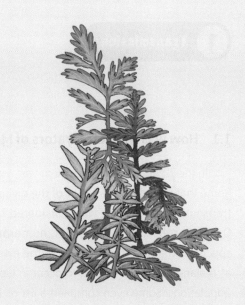

1 Transmission

1.1 How was the Perpetrators of Malaria Transmission Discovered?

In the 2nd and 3rd centuries BC, it was a widely held belief in ancient Greece and Rome that malaria was a result of the divine will, and the notion that "mosquitoes transmitted the disease was considered blasphemous and against God's will". Over the subsequent 100 years, numerous individuals began to suspect and speculate that the transmission of the disease was associated with mosquitoes, as malaria outbreaks tended to occur in wetland regions with abundant mosquito populations. Some even compiled a list of 19 accusations against mosquitoes, but due to a lack of convincing evidence, these accusations were ultimately laughed off and abandoned. Among these individuals, Dr. Patrick Manson, known as the "Verne of Pathology" and the "Mosquito Manson" (later called "Father of Tropical Medicine"), firmly believed that mosquitoes were the prime suspects in the transmission of malaria parasites. Manson encouraged Ronald Ross, a British doctor born in India who was 12 years his junior, to return to India where conditions were favorable for studying mosquitoes. He urged Ronald Ross to investigate which species of mosquitoes transmitted the disease and how it was transmitted? Upon returning to India, Ross, with his artistic temperament and distinctive personality, employed various methods to enable different species of mosquitoes to bite malaria-infected patients. For instance, such methods as placing mosquitoes within nets to bite bare-chested patients inside, directly placing newly hatched *Culex* and *Aedes* mosquitoes on patients, and then nurturing the blood-sucked mosquitoes, allowing them to hatch, and dissecting them one by one under a microscope were employed. After two years and three months of persistent and arduous observation, he finally discovered the oocyst of malaria parasites in the stomach cavity and walls of *Anopheles* mosquitoes, scientifically confirming the conjecture that mosquitoes transmitted malaria. However, Ross's curiosity was not satisfied. Ross even involved his 23-year-old son, who was studying in university at that time, in reverse comparison experiments. He made *Anopheles* mosquitoes that had sucked the blood of malaria patients directly bite the experimental subjects who had

1 传播

1.1 传播疟疾的凶手是怎么被发现的？

公元前二三世纪，在古希腊、古罗马，很长一段时期人们一直认为是神的意志产生了疟疾，而"蚊子传播疟疾的想法是亵渎神明、违反上帝意志的"。之后 100 多年间有许多人怀疑、猜测疟疾传播与蚊虫有关，因为疟疾流行地区总是在蚊虫较多的潮湿沼泽地带。还有人对蚊虫列出了足足 19 条罪状，但最终因为没有足够有说服力的证据，被人嘲笑而放弃。其中有个被人们称为"病理学上的凡尔纳""蚊虫曼森"的苏格兰医生帕特里克·曼森（Patrick Manson）爵士，其后被称为"热带医学之父"，他却坚信蚊虫是传播疟原虫的元凶。他鼓励比他小 12 岁、出生在印度的英国医生罗纳德·罗斯（Ronald Ross）回到有条件研究蚊虫的印度去研究是哪一种蚊虫传播疟疾的？又是通过什么样的方式传播的？有艺术气质和个性的罗纳德·罗斯回到印度后，用了许多方式让不同种类的蚊虫叮咬得病的疟疾患者。如把蚊虫放进蚊帐去叮咬躺在蚊帐内的赤膊的患者、将刚孵化出的库蚊、伊蚊直接放在患者身上叮咬等，然后把吸血后的蚊虫进行饲养、让其孵化，再在显微镜下一一解剖，经过 2 年 3 个月艰苦不懈的持久观察，终于在按蚊的胃腔和胃壁中发现了疟原虫卵囊，科学地证实了蚊虫传播疟疾的猜测。但他还不满足，甚至让其 23 岁正在读大学的儿子，参加了反向比较实验。他让吸过疟疾患者血的按蚊直接叮咬没有感染过疟疾的实验者，结果包括他儿子在内的实验者都感染上了疟疾，至此无可辩驳地证明了一种叫按蚊的蚊虫是传播疟疾的罪魁祸首。另外，他还在蚊虫的唾液中观察到了鸟类疟原虫。由此，罗纳

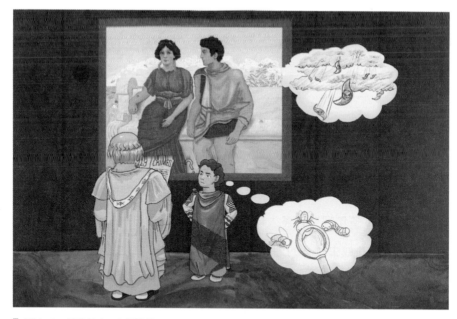

图 1-1　细数蚊虫 19 条罪状
Figure 1-1　19 Counts of Mosquitoes'Crimes

not been infected with malaria. As a result, all the experimental subjects, including his son, were infected with malaria, which irrefutably proved that *Anopheles* mosquitoes were the chief culprit in transmitting malaria. Furthermore, Ross observed avian malaria parasites in the saliva of mosquitoes. For his contributions to malaria research, particularly his confirmation that *Anopheles* mosquitoes were the vector to transmit malaria, Ross was awarded the Nobel Prize in Physiology or Medicine in 1902.

1.2　What do Malaria Parasites Look Like?

Malaria parasite is the pathogen that transmits malaria. Malaria parasite, a unicellular eukaryote, belongs to the genus *Plasmodium* within the phylum Apicomplexa, which is positioned at the top of the protozoan subkingdom. There are four main species of malaria parasites on human body , namely *Plasmodium vivax*, *Plasmodium falciparum*, *Plasmodium malariae* and *Plasmodium ovale*, *which* cause *Plasmodium vivax* malaria, *Plasmodium falciparum* malaria, *Plasmodium malariae* malaria and *ovale* malaria respectively. The development of malaria parasites necessitates the progression through two generations: asexual

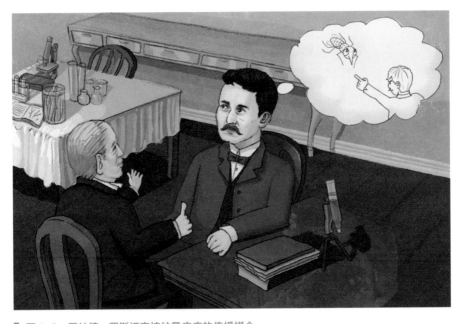

图 1-2　罗纳德·罗斯证实按蚊是疟疾的传播媒介
Figure 1-2　Ronald Ross Confirmed that *Anopheles* mosquito is the Vector of Malaria

德·罗斯因为证实按蚊是疟疾的传播媒介在探明疟疾病因上作出的贡献，荣获了 1902 年的诺贝尔生理学或医学奖。

1.2　疟原虫长啥样？

疟原虫是传播疟疾的病原体。疟原虫为单细胞真核生物，隶属于原虫动物亚界顶复门的疟原虫属。寄生于人体的疟原虫主要有 4 种，分别是间日疟原虫、恶性疟原虫、三日疟原虫和卵形疟原虫，它们分别引起间日疟、恶性疟、三日疟和卵形疟。疟原虫的发育需要经过无性生殖和有性生殖两个世代，这两个世代分别是在脊椎动物体内（主要是人）和媒介体内，如蚊虫（主要是按蚊）。4 种疟原虫的生活史基本相似，可以分为：红细胞外期、红细胞内期、配子生殖期和孢子增殖期。前两个时期在人体内完成，后两个时期在蚊虫体内完成。

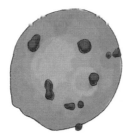

恶性疟原虫
Plasmodium falciparum

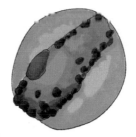

三日疟原虫
Plasmodium malariae

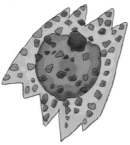

卵形疟原虫
Plasmodium ovale

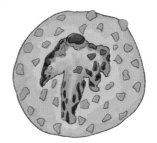

间日疟原虫
Plasmodium vivax

图 1-3　红细胞内疟原虫的形态
Figure 1-3　Morphology of Malaria Parasites in Erythrocytes

reproduction and sexual reproduction, which respectively take place within vertebrate hosts (principally humans) and intermediate hosts, such as mosquitoes (principally *Anopheles* spp.). The life cycles of the four species of malaria parasites are essentially similar, consisting of the extracellular phase, intraerythrocytic phase, gamete reproductive phase, and sporogenous phase. The first two phases are completed in humans, while the latter two are completed in mosquitoes.

The appearance of the four human malaria parasites in erythrocytes of peripheral blood differs. The different developmental phases of malaria parasites within erythrocytes can be classified into trophozoites, schizonts and gametocytes. Detecting malaria parasites within erythrocytes serves as the basis for diagnosing malaria and identifying insect species, and clinical laboratories typically utilize both thin and thick blood film methods on a single slide for examination.

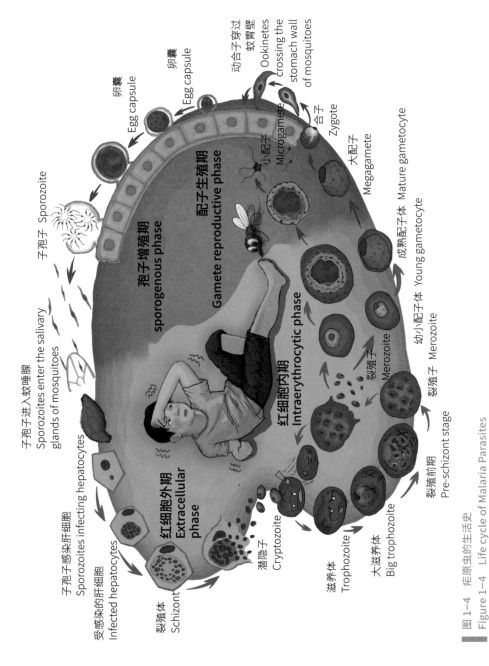

图 1-4　疟原虫的生活史
Figure 1-4　Life cycle of Malaria Parasites

子孢子进入蚊唾腺　子孢子 Sporozoite
Sporozoites enter the salivary
glands of mosquitoes

卵囊
Egg capsule

卵囊
Egg capsule

动合子穿过蚊胃壁
Ookinetes
crossing the
stomach wall
of mosquitoes

小配子 Microgamete

合子 Zygote

大配子 Megagamete

成熟配子体 Mature gametocyte

孢子增殖期 sporogenous phase

配子生殖期 Gamete reproductive phase

幼小配子体 Young gametocyte

裂殖子 Merozoite

子孢子感染肝细胞
Sporozoites infecting hepatocytes

红细胞外期 Extracellular phase

红细胞内期 Intraerythrocytic phase

裂殖子 Merozoite

受感染的肝细胞
Infected hepatocytes

潜隐子 Cryptozoite

裂殖体 Schizont

滋养体 Trophozoite

大滋养体 Big trophozoite

裂殖前期 Pre-schizont stage

4种人体疟原虫在末梢血液的红细胞内的样子是不一样的。疟原虫在红细胞内的不同发育阶段可分为滋养体、裂殖体和配子体。在红细胞内发现的疟原虫是确诊疟疾和鉴别虫种的依据，医院检验科通常采用在一张玻片上同时制作薄血膜和厚血膜的方法进行检查。

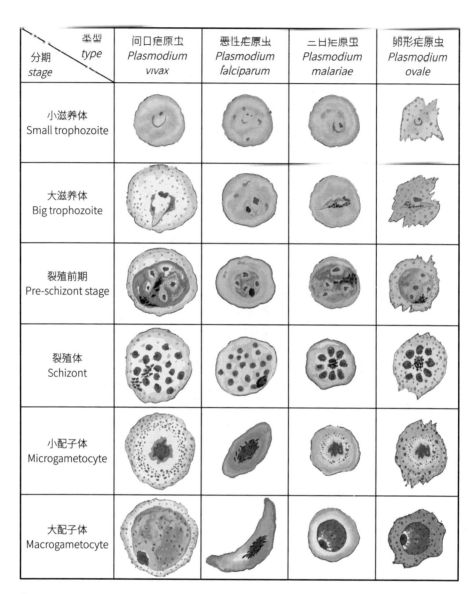

图 1-5　薄血膜下 4 种人体疟原虫形态
Figure 1-5　Morphology of Four Species of Human Malaria Parasites Under Thin Blood Smear

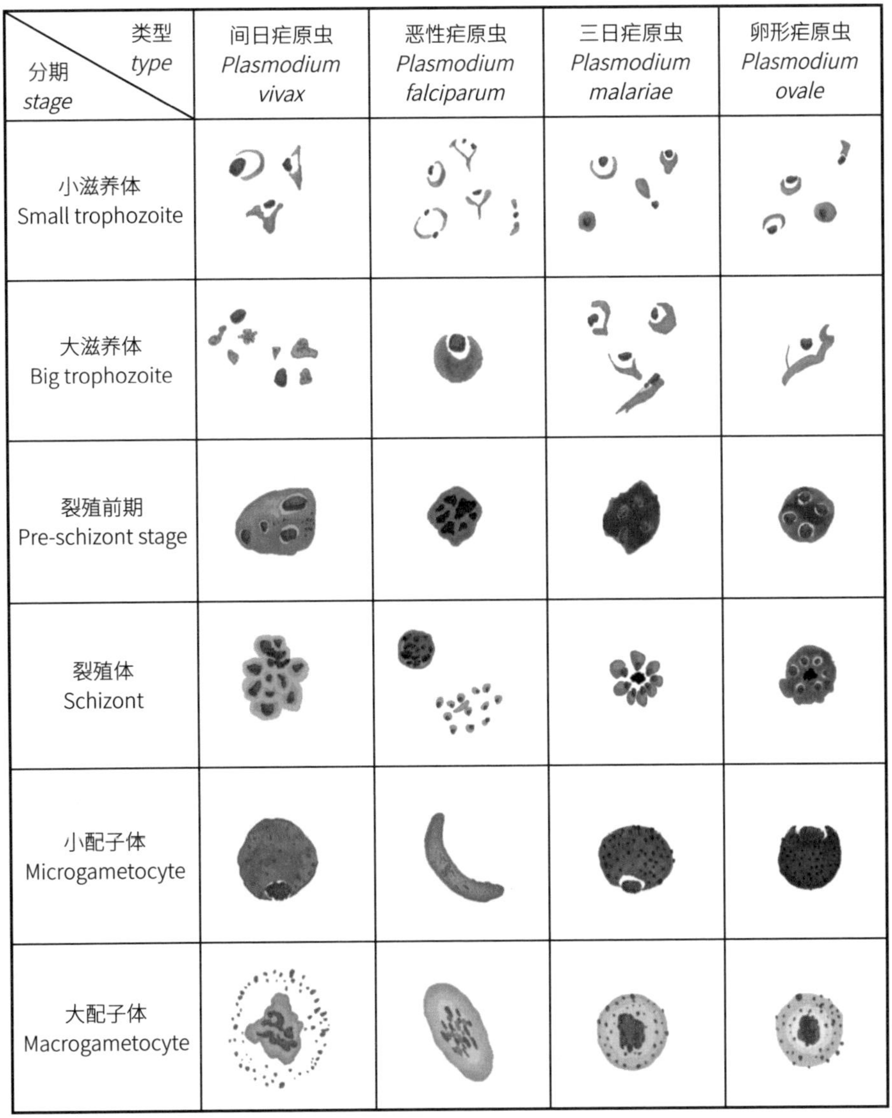

类型 type 分期 stage	间日疟原虫 *Plasmodium vivax*	恶性疟原虫 *Plasmodium falciparum*	三日疟原虫 *Plasmodium malariae*	卵形疟原虫 *Plasmodium ovale*
小滋养体 Small trophozoite				
大滋养体 Big trophozoite				
裂殖前期 Pre-schizont stage				
裂殖体 Schizont				
小配子体 Microgametocyte				
大配子体 Macrogametocyte				

图 1-6　厚血膜下 4 种人体疟原虫形态

Figure 1-6　Morphology of Four Species of Human Malaria Parasites Under Thick Blood Smear

1.2.1　Examination with Thin Blood Smear

1.2.1.1　*Plasmodium vivax*

The erythrocytes of parasitic *Plasmodium vivax* are generally 1.5 - 2 times larger than normal erythrocytes and also relatively light in color, with a few number of small bright red Schuffner's dots inside. Trophozoites are ring-shaped and relatively large, about 1/3 of the diameter of erythrocytes, with thick rings and mostly 1 nucleus. The volume of schizonts is larger than that of normal erythrocytes, and there are usually 16 merozoites, which are unevenly arranged, and 1 - 2 piles of malarial pigments gather. The microgametocytes are round, and their cytoplasm is light blue or light red, the nucleus is large and loose and often located in the center, and malarial pigments are scattered around the nucleus. The macrogametocytes are larger than normal erythrocytes, round or oval, and the nucleus is small, dense and purple-red, and malarial pigments are scattered in the cytoplasm.

1.2.1.2　*Plasmodium falciparum*

The erythrocytes of parasitic *Plasmodium falciparum* contain 3 - 5 Maurer's dots. Trophozoites are usually not seen in peripheral blood. The malarial pigments in the early phase are fine and golden, and will become lumpy and dark brown in the late phase. Mature trophozoites are also ring-shaped, with 2 nuclei. Schizonts are usually difficult to find in peripheral blood, because they are smaller than normal erythrocytes and dark brown. Therein, there are usually 18 - 26 merozoites, and the malarial pigments are lumpy and dark brown. Macrogametocytes are crescent-shaped, the nucleus is small and dense, dark red, and the cytoplasm is dark blue. The nuclear pigments are distributed loosely around the nucleus in the shape of sausage. Microgametocytes are sausage-shaped, with blunt ends, large and loose nucleus with reddish color, and malarial pigments are loosely distributed around the nucleus.

1.2.1.3　*Plasmodium malariae*

The erythrocytes of parasitic *Plasmodium malariae* show slender Simons' spots, which are lavender. Trophozoites are mostly mononuclear, and the malarial pigments are relatively coarse and dark brown, distributed along the edge of the polypide. The schizonts are smaller than the normal erythrocytes, with a round nucleus, and the malarial pigments are relatively coarse and often gather in the center. The macrogametocytes are smaller than normal erythrocytes, with round nuclei and a dark blue cytoplasm. The microgametocytes are usually smaller than normal erythrocytes, with large and loose nuclei and thick pigments scattered around the nuclei.

1.2.1 采用薄血膜的方法进行检查

1.2.1.1 间日疟原虫

间日疟原虫寄生的红细胞一般比正常的红细胞大 1.5 ～ 2 倍，颜色较浅，内部的薛氏点为鲜红色，数量少且小。滋养体呈环状体，较大，大约是红细胞直径的 1/3，环粗大，核大多是 1 个。裂殖体的体积大于正常的红细胞，其中的裂殖子通常为 16 个，且排列不均匀，疟色素聚集成 1 ～ 2 堆。小配子体成圆形，其胞浆为淡蓝或浅红色，核大且松散，常位于中央，疟色素散在核周围。大配子体的体积大于正常的红细胞，成圆形或者卵圆形，核小且致密，成紫红色，疟色素分散分布在胞浆中。

1.2.1.2 恶性疟原虫

恶性疟原虫寄生的红细胞含有 3 ～ 5 个紫红色的茂氏点。滋养体通常在外周血中看不到，早期的疟色素细小，金色，晚期结成块状，呈黑褐色。成熟的滋养体也呈环状，核常为 2 个。裂殖体通常在外周血中很难发现，因为它们小于正常的红细胞，成黑褐色。其中，裂殖子通常为 18 ～ 26 个，疟色素成团块状，呈黑褐色。大配子体成新月形，核小且致密，呈深红色，胞浆呈深蓝色，核色素成腊肠形松散分布于核周。小配子体成腊肠形，两端钝圆，核大且松散，呈淡红色，疟色素松散地分布于核周围。

1.2.1.3 三日疟原虫

三日疟原虫寄生的红细胞可见纤细的西门氏点，呈淡紫色。滋养体多为单核，疟色素较粗大，呈深褐色，沿虫体边缘分布。裂殖体小于正常的红细胞，核圆，疟色素较粗大，常聚集于中央。大配子体小于正常的红细胞，核成圆形，胞浆呈深蓝色。小配子体通常小于正常的红细胞，核大而松，色素散在核周，较粗大。

1.2.1.4 *Plasmodium ovale*

The front and back edges of erythrocytes of parasitic *Plasmodium ovale* are serrated and pale; Schuffner's dots appear earlier. Trophozoites are round or incomplete round, and the malarial pigments are thick and dark brown. The schizonts are similar to those of *Plasmodium Plasmodium* malaria, but the merozoites are slightly larger, usually eight. Macrogametocytes and microgametocytes are similar to those of *Plasmodium vivax* malaria, but smaller than normal erythrocytes.

1.2.2 Examination with Thick Blood Smear

1.2.2.1 *Plasmodium vivax*

A big trophozoite has a nucleus, and the polypide is relatively large. The cytoplasm is often broken into several pieces, during which yellow-green malarial pigments can be seen. There are 12 - 24 merozoites in a schizont. The gametocyte are round and the malarial pigments are yellow-green and shaped like a short rod.

1.2.2.2 *Plasmodium falciparum*

Big trophozoites are common in severe malaria, and are generally not found in peripheral blood. The polypide is irregular and round, and contain huge black lumps of malarial pigments. Schizonts are occasionally found in severe malaria, containing 18 - 36 merozoites. The macrogametocytes are crescent-shaped and the microgametocytes are ovoid; malarial pigments are golden yellow when scattered in fine particles, and black when aggregated into lumps.

1.2.2.3 *Plasmodium malariae*

A big trophozoite is banded or spherical, with one nucleus, deep blue cytoplasm and a large amount of malarial pigments. A schizont contains 6 - 12 merozoites. The gametocyte are round, and the malarial pigments are reddish brown and coarse sand-shaped.

1.2.2.4 *Plasmodium ovale*

A big trophozoite is usually round with irregular edges, and occasionally banded, with one nucleus and dark blue cytoplasm, containing 4 - 16 merozoites. The gametocyte are round, and the malarial pigments are yellowish brown and sand-shaped.

1.2.1.4　卵形疟原虫

卵形疟原虫寄生的红细胞前后边缘呈锯齿状，色淡；薛氏点出现较早。滋养体呈圆形或不整圆形，疟色素粗大，呈暗棕色。裂殖体与三日疟类似，但裂殖子稍大，通常为 8 个。大小配子体与间日疟类似，但小于正常红细胞。

1.2.2　采用厚血膜的方法进行检查

1.2.2.1　间日疟原虫

大滋养体有一个核，虫体较大，胞浆常断裂成数块，期内可见黄绿疟色素。裂殖体内含有 12 ～ 24 个裂殖子。配子体成圆形，疟色素呈黄绿色，类似短杆状。

1.2.2.2　恶性疟原虫

大滋养体常见于重症疟疾，一般不见于末梢血，虫体呈不规则圆形，其内有巨大的黑色疟色素团块。裂殖体偶见于重症疟疾，含有裂殖子 18 ～ 36 个。大配子体成新月形，小配子体成卵圆形；疟色素散为细粒时呈金黄色，聚集成团块后呈黑色。

1.2.2.3　三日疟原虫

大滋养体呈带状或球形，有一个核，胞浆蓝色甚深，含有大量疟色素。裂殖体有 6 ～ 12 个裂殖子。配子体呈圆形，疟色素呈棕褐色，粗砂粒状。

1.2.2.4　卵形疟原虫

大滋养体常为边缘不整齐的圆形，偶可呈带状，一个核，胞浆蓝色较深，有裂殖子 4 ～ 16 个。配子体呈圆形，疟色素呈黄褐色，沙粒状。

疟疾能在地球上消失吗？

014

Table 1-1　Identification Characteristics Commonly Used to Distinguish Four Species of Human Malaria Parasites

Insect species	Key Identification points	
	Thick blood Smear	Thin blood Smear
Plasmodium falciparum	The insect phase is consistent, and there are most of them are micro tropho-zoites	Erythrocytes do not swell
Plasmodium vivax	It can be observed that the cytoplasm is active in each phase, and a polypide close to the size of neutrophils can be seen	Infected erythrocytes can be observed to be larger than 1.5 times
Plasmodium malariae	It can be observed that the cytoplasm is strip-shaped in each phase, and chrysanthemum-shaped schizonts can be observed	Erythrocytes parasitized by malaria parasites do not swell or shrink
Plasmodium ovale	It can be observed that the cytoplasm is dense in each phase, and the polypide is smaller than Plasmodium vivax	The erythrocytes parasitized by malaria parasites are slightly larger, and the parasitized erythrocytes with long oval shape and serrated edge at one end can be observed
Negative blood Smear	If the typical morphology of malaria parasites (malaria pigment cytoplasm + nucleus) is not observed, it will be judged negative	

Characteristics of *Plasmodium vivax*: The erythrocytes parasitized by *Plasmodium vivax* are apparently swollen and faded. The Schuffner's spots are fine, small and numerous. A big trophozoite is ameboid. The vacuoles in the cytoplasm of the polypide are obvious. The pigment particles are short rod-shaped, fine and yellowish-brown.

Characteristics of *Plasmodium falciparum*: The erythrocytes parasitized by *Plasmodium falciparum* are normal in shape. The Maurer's dots are red, thick, obvious, and few in number; there is one or more red nuclei. Ring bodies are sometimes attached to the edge of erythrocytes, and multi-insect infection is quite common.

Characteristics of *Plasmodium malariae*: The morphology of erythrocytes parasitized by *Plasmodium malariae* is normal or slightly reduced. Big trophozoites are often banded (banded body). There is one relatively large nucleus and the cytoplasm is blue and relatively deep, with no obvious vacuoles. The pigment

表 1-1　常见的 4 种人体疟原虫的鉴别特点

虫种	关键鉴别要点	
	厚血膜	薄血膜
恶性疟原虫	虫期一致，且多为小滋养体	红细胞不胀大
间日疟原虫	各期可见，胞浆活跃，可观察到接近中性粒细胞大小的虫体	可观察到胀大 1.5 倍以上的被感染红细胞
三日疟原虫	各期可见，胞浆呈条状，可观察到菊花状裂殖体	被原虫寄生的红细胞不胀大或缩小
卵形疟原虫	各期可见，胞浆致密，虫体与间日疟原虫比较偏小	被原虫寄生的红细胞略胀大，可观察到长椭圆形、一端边缘呈锯齿状的被寄生红细胞
阴性血片	若观察不到典型的原虫形态（疟色素 + 胞浆 + 核）则判阴性	

间日疟原虫的特点：被间日疟原虫寄生的红细胞明显胀大，褪色。薛氏点细小，数多。大滋养体呈阿米巴样。虫体胞质内空泡明显。色素颗粒为短杆状，较细，呈黄褐色。

恶性疟原虫的特点：被恶性疟原虫寄生的红细胞形态正常。茂氏点为红色，粗大，明显。有 1 个或多个红色的核。环状体有时贴于红细胞边缘，多虫感染较常见。

三日疟原虫的特点：被三日疟原虫寄生的红细胞形态正常或稍缩小。大滋养体常呈带状（带状体）。核一个，较大，细胞质呈蓝色，较深，空泡不明显。色素颗粒粗大，成砂粒状，深褐色，一般染色下红细胞中无点彩，浓缩时可见紫蓝色点彩，称西门氏点。

卵形疟原虫的特点：被卵形疟原虫寄生的红细胞稍胀大或不胀大，有伞矢状边缘。早期出现薛氏点或詹姆斯点，明显粗大。虫体无明显伪足，成熟的虫体小于正常红细胞。色素颗粒粗大，成砂粒状，深褐色。

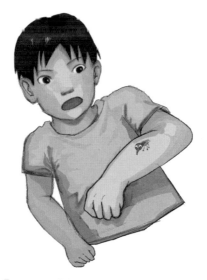

图 1-7　超级杀手——蚊子
Figure 1-7　Super Killer — Mosquitoes

particles are coarse and sand-shaped, dark brown, and there are no basophilic stippling under general dyeing. When concentrated, purple-blue basophilic stippling can be seen, referred to as Simon's spots.

Characteristics of *Plasmodium ovale*: The erythrocytes parasitized by *Plasmodium ovale* swell slightly or not, with umbrella sagittal edges. Schuffner's dots or James's spots appear in the early phase, obviously coarse. The polypide has no obvious pseudopodia, and a mature polypide is smaller than normal erythrocytes. The pigment particles are coarse, sand-shaped and dark brown.

1.3　Case 1　Can Mosquitoes Kill People Through Malaria Parasites?

You know what? Killing human beings is a matter of minutes for me! "Top Nemesis" and "Top Predator" are the most proud titles that human beings have given me. I try my means to control at least 700,000 lives every year through various small arms, such as viruses, bacteria and parasites! I am the super killer.

It's even a piece of cake to kill people simply with the use of malaria parasites. 600 000 lives died at my hands in 2020 alone. Remember? When Mr. Li returned to China from Africa, he had a fever and a little diarrhea. He thought it was a cold, and he took some cold and anti-fever drugs himself, rather than take it seriously.

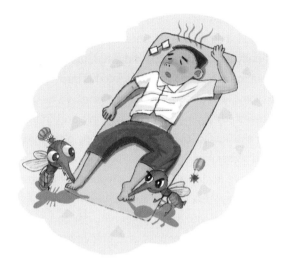

图 1-8 蚊子传播疟原虫
Figure 1-8 Transmission of Malaria Parasites by Mosquitoes

1.3 案例 1 蚊子能通过疟原虫杀死人吗？

你知道吗？杀死人类对我们蚊子来说是分分钟的事！顶级克星、顶级掠食者是人类赋予我最得意的称呼。我用尽各种手段，带上各种小武器，如病毒、细菌、寄生虫等，每年至少把控着 70 多万条人命！我就是超级杀手。

用疟原虫来杀人更是小事一桩，仅 2020 年一年就有 60 多万条命丧于我手。还记得吗？那次李先生从非洲回到中国，发烧了，还有点拉肚子，以为是感冒，就自己吃了点感冒退烧药，没当一回事，结果直接昏迷在自动驾驶汽车上，送到医院时直接卧倒，不省人事！医生查来查去，最后查出是我做的手脚，我就轻轻地叮了他一下，直接把我体内的小妖魔——疟原虫输入他的体内。你看到了吧，你们不马上用点撒手锏把小妖魔杀死，所有人类都顶不住，都是我的手下败将，我所向披靡，嘚瑟着呢。在非洲，或者各种我喜欢待的地方，被我叮咬，"吻一下"太普通不过了，你们都不把我当回事，有

As a result, he directly lost consciousness in the self-driving car, and when he was taken to the hospital, he fell down directly, unconscious! The doctor conducted several examinations and finally it turned out that I did it. I just bit him gently and directly put the little demon in me — malaria parasites into his body. You see, if you don't kill the little demon with some killer at once, all human beings will be overwhelmed, and all of them will be my defeated opponents. I am invincible and smug about it. It is quite common to be bitten and "kissed" by me in Africa or any place I like to stay. You don't take me seriously, and sometimes you may not even know that I secretly sucked your blood. Don't underestimate my lethality. I have a hidden secret weapon, which will kill you when it enters your body. Also, I like to "collect honey" in various populations, and I like different tastes. I bother you, then bother him, her and it, and scatter my little demon into the "universe". I am never tired of it, enjoying my joy ... However, my life is also rather cheap. So long as you see through me, or don't let me take advantage of the loopholes to bite you and sneak up on you, I'll run away on my own.

1.4 Which Kind of Mosquito Likes Malaria Parasites?

Female *Anopheles* mosquitoes are the most fond of malaria parasites, and there are more than 400 species of *Anopheles* mosquitoes in 6 subgenera known in the world, of which there are around 35 important malaria vectors. Among them more than 60 known species of *Anopheles* mosquitoes in China, there are 4 main malaria vectors, including *Anopheles sinensis* and *Anopheles anthropophagus* of subgenus *Anopheles*, and *Anopheles minimus* and *Anopheles dirus* of subgenus Cellia.

Anopheles sinensis sucks both human and animal blood and prefers to suck animal blood. It is the main or only vector of *Plasmodium vivax* in the plain area north of latitude 34° in China. It belongs to semi-domestic mosquito species. Adult mosquitoes like to live on the wall 1 - 2 meters above the ground in cattle houses, while adult mosquitoes in the wild like to live in dark and humid hidden places or paddy fields. The number of its population changes seasonally, which is closely associated with the temperature, rainfall and farming system in various places. For instance, they will appear all year round in places south of 27 ° north latitude; while at 28 ° - 32 ° north latitude, it is semi-overwintering in winter; in the north of 33° north latitude, it is in a state of complete wintering. Larvae like to live in paddy fields, ponds, puddles, reed ponds, swamps and depressions and water holes, etc. In regions where residents have relatively poor conditions to prevent and control mosquitoes and maintain the habits of sleeping in the open in summer and autumn,

时候可能都不知道被我偷偷吸了血。不要小看我的杀伤力，我有隐藏的秘密武器，进入你体内可是会要你小命的。还有啊，我喜欢在各种种群中"采采蜜"，喜欢不同的口味，惹惹你，再惹惹他、她、它，把我体内的小妖魔撒向"宇宙"。我乐此不疲，欢快着我的欢快……不过，我的命也相当廉价，只要你识破我，或者不让我钻空子叮咬你，偷袭你，我也就自己灰溜溜地逃了。

1.4　哪种蚊子喜欢疟原虫？

雌性按蚊最喜欢疟原虫，全世界已知按蚊有 6 亚属 400 多种，其中重要的传疟媒介有 35 种左右。在中国已知的 60 余种按蚊中，主要传疟媒介有 4 种，包括按蚊亚属的中华按蚊、嗜人按蚊，塞蚊亚属的微小按蚊和大劣按蚊。

中华按蚊，兼吸人、畜血而偏爱吸畜血。在北纬 34°以北的平原地区，它是我国主要的或唯一的间日疟传播媒介。它属于半家栖蚊种，成蚊喜欢栖息于牛房离地面 1 ～ 2m 高的墙壁上，野外的成蚊则喜欢栖息于阴暗潮湿的隐蔽场所或稻田里。其种群数量有季节性变动，与各地的气温、雨量和耕作制度有密切关系，如：在北纬 27°以南的地方，它们全年都会出现；在北纬 28°～ 32°，冬季它们呈半越冬的状态；而在北纬 33°以北，它们则处于完全越冬状态。幼虫喜欢生活在稻田、池塘、水坑、芦苇塘、沼泽和洼地积水等处。在居民防蚊条件较差、夏秋季有露宿习惯的地区，由于与人接触的机会增加且种群数量大，常导致疟疾流行或暴发。

嗜人按蚊（也称雷氏按蚊）为恶性疟的主要传播媒介。它们属于家栖蚊种，喜欢吸人血，主要栖息在人类居住的房间，也喜欢栖息于牛房及其他有禽类、畜类的房间里。幼虫喜欢生活在清凉、缓慢流动和有植物遮阴的水体中，如：沟渠、稻田、茭白田和池塘等处。它们一般在每年的 8 ～ 10 月份出

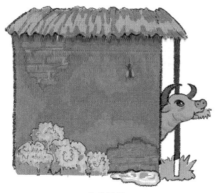

中华按蚊
Anopheles sinensis

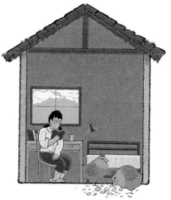

嗜人按蚊
Anopheles anthropophagus

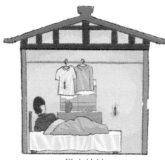

微小按蚊
Anopheles minimus

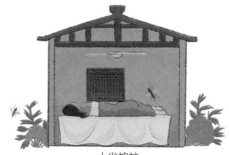

大劣按蚊
Anopheles dirus

图 1-9   四种传疟媒介
Figure 1-9   Four Vectors of Malaria

malaria endemics or outbreaks often occur due to increased contact with people and large numbers of populations.

Anopheles anthropophagus (*Anopheles lesteri*) are the main vector of (*Plasmodium falciparum*) malaria. They belong to domestic mosquito species and prefer to suck human blood. These mosquitoes principally inhabit human houses, and also prefer to inhabit cattle houses and other houses with poultry and livestock. Larvae prefer to live in cool and slow-moving water bodies shaded by plants, e.g., ditches, paddy fields, water bamboo fields and ponds, etc. *Anopheles anthropophagus* generally appear from August to October every year and will also appear in June and July in the central and southern regions; they often overwinter as eggs or adult mosquitoes.

Anopheles minimus, a domestic mosquito species, prefer to suck cattle blood.

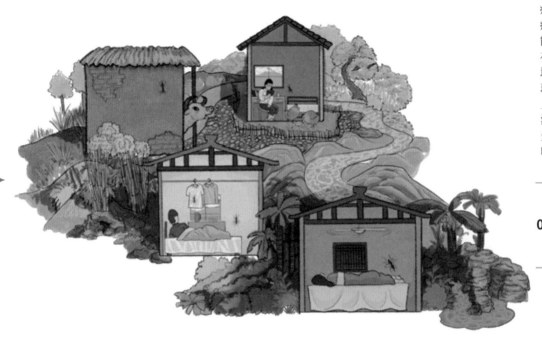

现，在中南部地区也会在 6、7 月份出现；常以卵或成蚊的形式越冬。

微小按蚊属于家栖蚊种，偏爱吸牛血。它们主要分布于我国北纬 33°以南的山丘地区，在北纬 25°以南地区最为普遍。它们为疟疾的重要媒介之一。成蚊喜欢栖息在室内离地面 1～2m 高的墙壁上或悬挂的衣服上，野外的成蚊喜欢栖息在石洞、竹丛和草丛等地；幼虫喜欢生活在有阳光、半遮阴、水流缓慢、水质清澈的溪沟里，尤其是有杂草的岸边。在海南，它们通常出现在雨季前的 3～5 月份；而在云南等地它们会出现在雨季后的 9～10 月份；常以幼虫期越冬。

大劣按蚊，为热带丛林型按蚊，主要分布于海南，在云南南部和广西西南部也有分布，为海南山地森林地区重要的传疟媒介。它们属于野栖蚊种，喜欢吸人血，夜间入房吸饱血后，稍作停留，便飞向屋外，白天很难在屋内找到它们。幼虫主要生活在有良好遮阴的山涧、岩石、小溪浅洼和石穴积水

These mosquitoes are principally distributed in hilly regions south of 33° north latitude in China, and are most prevalent in the area south of 25° north latitude. They are one of the important vectors of malaria. Adult mosquitoes prefer to inhabit indoor walls 1 - 2 meters above the ground or hanging clothes, while adult mosquitoes in the wild prefer to inhabit caves, bamboo bushes and grasslands, etc. Larvae prefer to live in sunny, semi-shaded, slow-water flowing, clear-water gullies, and mostly on the banks with weeds. In Hainan, they tend to appear in March to May before the rainy season; in Yunnan and other places, they will appear in September to October after the rainy season; they often overwinter in larval phase.

Anopheles dirus, a species of tropical jungle *Anopheles* mosquito, are not only chiefly distributed in Hainan, but also in southern Yunnan and southwestern Guangxi. They are important vectors of malaria in the mountainous forest regions of Hainan. They belong to the wild mosquito species, and like to suck human blood. After entering the house at night and being full of blood, they will stop for a while and fly outside. It is difficult to find them in the house during the day. Larvae principally live in well-shaded mountain streams, rocks, shallow depressions in streams and stagnant water in caves. Adult mosquitoes often live in caves, bushes and weeds, particularly in caves. They usually appear from August to October after the rainy season every year.

1.5　How to Carry out Prevention and Control Measures in High Endemic Regions?

Tips

(1) *Anopheles dirus* is strongly capable of transmitting malaria.

(2) Simply treating malaria patients and reducing the sources of infection can only temporarily reduce the prevalence of malaria in the local area, but it cannot eradicate the sources of infection, making the malaria endemic prone to rebounds.

(3) The sole reliance on indoor insecticide residual spraying for the prevention and control of *Anopheles dirus* is also insufficient.

(4) Malaria-endemic regions with *Anopheles dirus* as the main transmission vector need to be divided into different regions based on the prevalence of *Anopheles dirus* and the incidence of malaria, implementing measures according to local conditions and providing targeted guidance.

中。成蚊常栖息于石洞、灌木丛和杂草丛中，尤其喜欢栖息在石洞中。它们通常在每年雨季后的 8～10 月份出现。

1.5　如何在高流行地区开展疟疾防控？

小提示

（1）大劣按蚊传播疟疾能力强。

（2）单纯通过治疗疟疾患者，减少传染源的防治办法只能暂时降低当地疟疾流行程度，无法消灭传染源，疟疾疫情易反弹。

（3）单靠室内杀虫剂滞留喷洒对大劣按蚊的防制效果也不佳。

（4）以大劣按蚊为主要媒介的疟疾流行区需要依据大劣按蚊流行程度和疟疾发病率进行分区，因地制宜，分类指导。

大劣按蚊是一种高效的疟疾传播媒介，我国主要分布于海南，广西壮族自治区的西南部、云南省的南部和西藏自治区的东南部等地区亦有少量分布。海南省经过大量实践发现在以大劣按蚊为主要媒介的疟疾流行区仅通过治疗疟疾患者减少传染源的措施虽能暂时降低当地疟疾流行程度，但由于媒介按蚊的存在，无法彻底清除残存传染源，疟疾可以在短期内恢复传播；同时由于大劣按蚊为野栖蚊种，白天极少栖息于室内，只在黄昏或夜间才飞到居住地附近，于吸血前后停栖于屋檐下或室外灌木丛、草丛中，在室内的停栖时间很短，极少停留在室内过夜，因此仅靠室内杀虫剂滞留喷洒对其防制效果不佳；仅清除居民点周围的灌木丛，虽然可使大劣按蚊滋生地直接暴露于阳光下，有效地降低其幼虫密度，控制疟疾的流行，但部分村庄或因居民较少无力清理环境，或因周围地势陡峭，清理后的场地不宜于耕种，难以管理维持，杂草灌木很快又重新生长，幼虫迅速重新滋生。

20 世纪 50 年代海南省针对以大劣按蚊为主要媒介的山林地带疟疾流行

Anopheles dirus is an efficient vector for malaria transmission, primarily distributed in Hainan Island, with smaller quantities found in the southwestern part of Guangxi Zhuang Autonomous Region, the southern part of Yunnan Province, and the southeastern part of the Xizang Autonomous Region in china. After extensive practice in Hainan Province, it was found that although the measure of solely treating malaria patients and reducing sources of infection in malaria-endemic regions with *Anopheles dirus* as the main vector can temporarily reduce the prevalence of malaria in the local area, it cannot totally eradicate the remaining sources of infection due to the presence of vector *Anopheles* mosquitoes, making malaria susceptible to resumption of transmission in the short term. Simultaneously, due to *Anopheles dirus* being a wild-inhabiting mosquito species, it rarely shelters indoors during the day and only flies to residential regions near dusk or night. It stops resting under eaves or in outdoor shrubs and grasses before and after blood sucking, with a short indoor resting phase and rarely staying indoors overnight. Therefore, the sole indoor residual spraying of insecticides has insufficient prevention and control effects on it. While solely clearing the bushes around residential regions can expose the breeding sites of *Anopheles dirus* to direct sunlight, effectively reducing their larvae density and controlling the prevalence of malaria, some villages may face difficulties in cleaning the environment due to a smaller population or steep surrounding terrain. The cleared regions are not suitable for farming, making it difficult to manage and maintain, and weeds and bushes quickly regrow, leading to a rapid resurgence of larvae.

In the 1950s, Hainan Province took comprehensive prevention and control measures in malaria-endemic regions dominated by *Anopheles dirus* as the main transmission vector, combining the unique ecological habits of *Anopheles dirus* and implementing some practical prevention and control measures. Prior to 1982, indoor residual spraying of mosquito-killing insecticides along with mass drug administration for local population were conducted twice a year. The incidence of malaria in the vast rural regions gradually decreased from 3,490 cases per 10,000 in 1957 to 42 cases per 10,000 in 1982. Besides implementing the aforementioned routine anti-malaria measures, some mountainous regions covered by dense forests, in conjunction with local production and construction needs, cleared dense forests near residential regions in a planned and step-by-step manner, planted economic crops, promptly reduced the regional incidence of malaria and maintained it at a low level.

区，除坚持采用综合性防控措施外，还结合大劣按蚊特殊的生态习性与实际可能，采取了一些可行的防控措施。1982 年以前，每年进行两次灭蚊药物的室内滞留喷洒和全民药物治疗；广大农村的发病率从 1957 年的 3490 人次 / 万逐步下降到 1982 年的 42 人次 / 万。一些丛林覆盖的山区除开展上述常规抗疟措施外，还结合当地生产和建设需求，逐年有计划、有步骤地清除居民居住地附近的密林，种植经济作物，迅速降低区域疟疾发病率，且稳定在较低水平。

1982 年起，经过多年的综合防治后，海南省不少地区发病率下降，部分地区开发后生态环境发生了改变。为此，海南省积极开展疟疾病例监测，根治现症患者和带虫者；加强山区流动人口管理，给予预防药，加强个人防护；在发病率较高的地区实施全民服药和杀虫剂室内滞留喷洒，开发和清理村庄周围环境，破坏媒介按蚊滋生栖息条件等基本防治策略后，对以大劣按蚊为主要媒介的疟疾流行区重新进行分区，因地制宜地实施策略并分类指导。对于居民发病率已降到 1% 以下且未发现大劣按蚊的地区，停止杀虫剂室内滞留喷洒，重点做好现症患者的及时发现和治疗工作。对于大劣按蚊数量较少而微小按蚊数量相对较多、发病率在 1% ～ 5% 的地区，每年用杀虫剂室内滞留喷洒 1 ～ 2 次，并对个别发病较高的村庄进行全民服药，同时加强疟疾监测。对于大劣按蚊长年存在且数量较多、发病率一般在 5% ～ 10% 的村庄，每年仍用杀虫剂室内滞留喷洒 1 ～ 2 次，进行全民治疗 2 次。采取以上针对性防控措施后，以大劣按蚊为主要传疟媒介的海南黎族苗族自治州，居民疟疾发病率继续稳步下降，1982 年为 77 人次／万，1983 年为 50 人次 / 万，1984 年为 48 人次／万。

Since 1982, after years of comprehensive prevention and control, the incidence of malaria has decreased in many regions of Hainan Province, and the ecological environment has changed in some developed regions. To this end, Hainan Province has actively monitored malaria cases, effected a radical cure for existing patients and carriers, strengthened the management of migratory populations in mountainous regions, provided prophylactic medication, and enhanced personal protection. After implementing basic prevention and control strategies, including mass drug administration and indoor residual spraying of insecticides, developing and clearing the surrounding environments of villages, and destroying breeding and resting conditions for *Anopheles* mosquitoes in some regions with a relatively high incidence of malaria, malaria-endemic regions with *Anopheles dirus* as the main vector were redivided into different regions for implementing measures according to local conditions and providing targeted guidance. In regions where the incidence of malaria among residents had dropped below 1% and no *Anopheles dirus* had been detected, indoor residual spraying of insecticides was halted, and the focus was placed on timely detection and treatment of existing patients. In regions where there were few *Anopheles dirus* but relatively abundant *Anopheles minimus*, with the incidence ranging from 1% to 5%, indoor residual spraying of insecticides was conducted annually for 1 to 2 times, mass drug administration was implemented in individual villages with a higher incidence of malaria, and malaria surveillance was strengthened as well. In villages where *Anopheles dirus* was present throughout the year and in large numbers, with an incidence of malaria generally ranging from 5% to 10%, indoor residual spraying of insecticides was still used annually for 1 to 2 times, and mass drug administration was conducted twice. After adopting these targeted prevention and control measures, the incidence of malaria among residents of the Hainan Li and Miao Autonomous Prefecture, where *Anopheles dirus* was the main vector, continued to decline steadily. In 1982, the incidence was 77 cases per 10,000, dropping to 50 cases per 10,000 in 1983 and further to 48 cases per 10,000 in 1984.

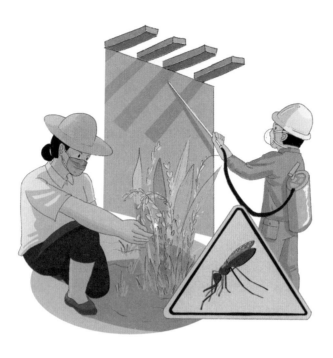

图 1-10　杀虫剂室内滞留喷洒防控大劣按蚊
Figure 1-10　Indoor Residual Spraying of Insecticides to Prevent and Control *Anopheles dirus*

2 Symptoms

2.1 What are the General Clinical Symptoms of Malaria?

Tips

(1) In cases of patients with a relevant epidemiological exposure history (i.e., residing in malaria-endemic regions or traveling to such regions) presenting with fever (temperature ≥ 37.5° C), malaria should be considered.

(2) Apart from fever, the initial symptoms of malaria can include tachycardia, tachypnea, shivering, discomfort, fatigue, sweating, headache, dry cough, anorexia, nausea, vomiting, abdominal pain, diarrhea, arthralgia, and myalgia, among other non-specific symptoms.

(3) If a patient has symptoms consistent with malaria and the examination result of malaria parasites is positive, malaria can be diagnosed.

After being bitten by an infected female *Anopheles* mosquito, infected individuals usually experience an asymptomatic period of 2 to 4 weeks, medically known as the incubation period. However, symptoms can appear as early as 7 days after the bite, depending on the species of malaria parasite.

Most *Plasmodium falciparum* infections manifest within 1 month. Those who have previously contracted malaria may exhibit a longer incubation period. *Plasmodium vivax* and *Plasmodium ovale* are recurrent types of malaria parasite, with an incubation period of approximately 2 weeks. However, several months after the initial infection, patients can become ill due to the activation of dormant parasites remaining in the liver. The incubation period for *Plasmodium malariae* is around 18 days, but asymptomatic infections may persist for several years.

When erythrocytes infected with malaria parasites rupture, they will release a malaria parasite form known as merozoites, which cause fever and other clinical manifestations of malaria. Apart from fever, the initial symptoms of malaria also include tachycardia, tachypnea, shivering, discomfort, fatigue, sweating, headache,

2 症 状

2.1 疟疾的一般临床症状有哪些?

> **小提示**
>
> (1) 对于有相关流行病学暴露史（即居住在疟区或前往疟区旅行）的发热患者（体温 ≥ 37.5℃），应考虑疟疾。
>
> (2) 疟疾的初始症状除发热还包括心动过速、呼吸过速、寒战、不适、乏力、出汗、头痛、干咳、厌食、恶心、呕吐、腹痛、腹泻、关节痛和肌痛等各种非特异性症状。
>
> (3) 如果患者有符合疟疾的症状且疟原虫检查结果为阳性，则可以确诊疟疾。

被感染的雌性按蚊叮咬后，感染者通常会有 2～4 周的时间没有症状，医学上称为潜伏期，但最快也有叮咬后 7 日就出现症状的，具体长短往往取决于疟原虫种类。

大多数恶性疟原虫感染者在 1 个月内出现临床表现。以往感染过疟疾的人更有可能出现较长的潜伏期。间日疟原虫和卵形疟原虫是可复发的疟原虫类型，它们的潜伏期约为 2 周，但在初始感染后数月，患者可能会因肝内休眠子激活而发病。三日疟原虫的潜伏期约为 18 日，但无症状感染可能会持续好几年。

被疟原虫感染的红细胞破裂时会释放出一种称为裂殖子的疟原虫，并导致发热及疟疾的其他临床表现。疟疾的初始症状除了发热，还包括心动过速、呼吸过速、寒战、不适、乏力、出汗、头痛、干咳、厌食、恶心、呕吐、腹痛、腹泻、关节痛和肌痛。医生检查可以发现贫血，并且在肋下可触及脾脏。没有免疫力的急性疟疾患者中，数日后可触及肿大脾脏。对于这类患者，他

dry cough, anorexia, nausea, vomiting, abdominal pain, diarrhea, arthralgia, and myalgia. The doctor can detect anaemia during an examination, and the spleen can be palpated below the ribs. In acute malaria patients without immunity, the spleen can be felt enlarged several days after the onset of symptoms. For such patients, there is often no anaemia in the early phases of their clinical course, so malaria should not be ruled out solely based on the absence of anaemia.

Although *Plasmodium falciparum* is the most pathogenic, it is usually impossible to determine the species of malaria infection solely based on clinical manifestations. In the early phases of malaria infection, fever is usually irregular, and the patient's temperature may rise above 40°C, accompanied by tachycardia and delirium. In the later phases of infection, when infected erythrocytes rupture, schizonts ruptured and merozoites will be released from the erythrocytes. Accompanying this regular rupture and release, *Plasmodium vivax* malaria attacks are more likely to have regular intervals. With the improvement of medical diagnosis and treatment, the phenomenon of periodic fever (colloquially known as "suffering from malaria") appearing in the late phases of infection is now rare.

2.2　Case 2　Why do Malaria Fever and Chills Alternate in Intensity?

Mr. Zhang, in his 50s, is a contracted overseas worker sent by his company to work in Africa in the past two years. Recently, he returned to China for a family visit and felt a bit chilled after arriving home. Not paying much attention to it, he continued with his daily activities. However, two days later, his temperature kept rising, and he began to experience headaches and vomiting. At the urging of his wife, Mr. Zhang went to the emergency department of a local hospital for a preliminary examination. No significant abnormalities were detected, so the doctor gave him some antipyretic drugs and oral antibiotics. But his condition didn't improve; instead, he started to experience confusion, delirium, and incontinence, etc. These symptoms made Mr. Zhang's family anxious, and they sent him to the emergency department immediately. After learning that Mr. Zhang had just returned from Africa, the emergency doctor urgently invited an infectious diseases specialist for a consultation. After relevant examinations, Mr. Zhang was diagnosed with severe *Plasmodium falciparum* malaria. He was immediately given anti-malaria medication and recovered from the critical condition.

们的临床病程早期常无贫血，不应仅凭没有贫血而排除疟疾。

虽然恶性疟原虫致病力最强，但通常不可能单凭临床表现来确定疟疾感染种类。在疟疾感染的早期，发热通常并无规律，患者的体温可能升至40°C以上，还可能伴有心动过速和谵妄。在感染较后期，感染红细胞破裂，同时发生裂殖体破裂且裂殖子从红细胞释放。伴随这种规律性的破裂和释放，间日疟的发作更常具有规律间隔性。随着诊疗水平的提升，这种感染晚期才出现的周期性发热（俗称"打摆子 ①"）的体征现已少见。

2.2　案例2　为什么疟疾发热与发冷呈一张一弛？

老张50来岁，是公司外派的劳务输出人员，近两年一直在非洲工作。近期他回国探亲，到家后自觉有些感冒着凉，一开始也没有在意，继续日常生活。但2天后他的体温越来越高，并出现了头痛、呕吐等症状。在老张媳妇的催促下，他到当地医院急诊部就诊，初步检查没有发现明显的异常，医生开了一些退热药和口服抗生素治疗。但其症状非但没有改善，还出现了意识模糊、说胡话、尿失禁等症状，这可急坏了老张一家人，赶紧将老张送到了医院的急诊部。急诊医生在得知老张最近才从非洲回国的情况后，赶紧请来了感染科医生会诊，经过相关检查最终确诊为重症恶性疟，立即给予特效的抗疟药治疗和抢救后才转危为安。

老张和家人在感谢医务人员的同时，对于疟疾还是产生了些许疑问：疟疾不就是"打摆子"吗？而老张本人并没有出现相应的典型表现，为什么自己的疟疾没有出现"打摆子"就一下子这么严重了呢？感染科的王医生解释到，老张得的是恶性疟，而以前在我国疟疾流行区以间日疟的流行为主，两者的表现各不相同，相比恶性疟，间日疟的发作更常具有规律间隔期，俗称"打摆子"。

---

① 当地称疟疾为打摆子。

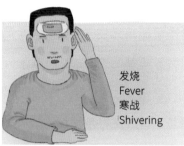
发烧
Fever
寒战
Shivering

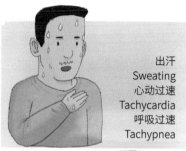
出汗
Sweating
心动过速
Tachycardia
呼吸过速
Tachypnea

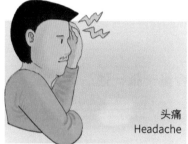
头痛
Headache

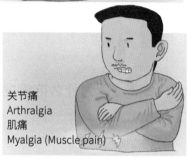
关节痛
Arthralgia
肌痛
Myalgia (Muscle pain)

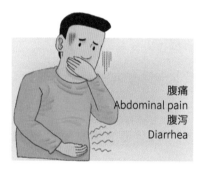
腹痛
Abdominal pain
腹泻
Diarrhea

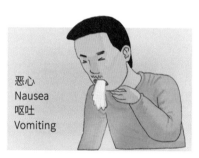
恶心
Nausea
呕吐
Vomiting

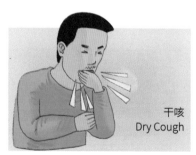
干咳
Dry Cough

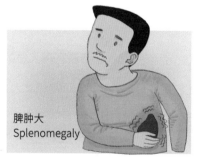
脾肿大
Splenomegaly

图 2-1　疟疾的临床表现
Figure 2-1　Clinical Symptoms of Malaria

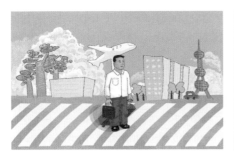

老张从非洲打工回国探亲
Mr. Zhang returns to his hometown in China for a family visit after spending time working in Africa.

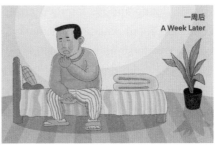

一周后自觉有感冒症状
One week later, he notices symptoms of a cold.

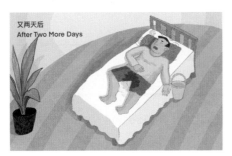

又两天后出现发热、头痛和呕吐症状
Two days later, he develops fever, headache, and vomiting.

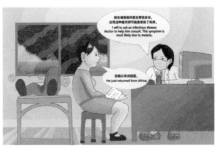

家人送老张紧急就医
His family rushes him to the emergency department of local hospital for treatment.

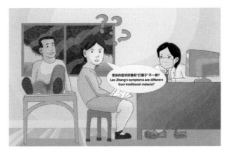

确诊感染重症恶性疟
He is diagnosed with severe *Plasmodium falciparum* malaria.

图 2-2　回国探亲人员感染疟疾与国内常见疟疾症状不一样吗？
Figure 2-2　Do the Symptoms of Malaria Infection Differ for Returnees Visiting Relatives from abroad Compared to the Common Malaria Symptoms in China?

Mr. Zhang and his family thanked the medical staff while expressing their confusion about malaria: isn't malaria defined as "suffering from malaria"? They couldn't understand why Mr. Zhang's malaria was so severe without showing the typical symptoms of "suffering from malaria". Infectious diseases specialist Dr. Wang explained that Mr. Zhang had infected with *Plasmodium falciparum* malaria, which is different from the *Plasmodium vivax* malaria that was previously dominant in malaria-endemic regions of China; the manifestations of the two are distinct; *Plasmodium vivax* malaria tends to have more regular intervals than *Plasmodium falciparum* malaria, i.e., "suffering from malaria."

2.3 What are the Clinical Symptoms of Special Types of Malaria?

Tips

Special clinical symptoms are chiefly caused by individual factors.

Dr. Wang further explained that Mr. Zhang's confusion and talking nonsense were Symptoms of cerebral malaria. Cerebral malaria is a brain disease characterized by impaired consciousness, delirium, and epileptic seizures. Patients may gradually develop the disease or experience sudden onset after seizures. The severity depends upon various factors such as the pathogen's pathogenicity, host immune response, and the interval between symptom onset and treatment initiation. Compared to local residents in African malaria-endemic regions, those who have recently traveled to Africa among adults, are more susceptible to cerebral malaria due to a lack of immunity, but cerebral malaria is more common in children among locals. Cerebral malaria is extremely dangerous, as it can progress rapidly to coma and even death. Thus, prompt assessment and treatment are necessary after observing cerebral malaria symptoms, otherwise, it is almost always fatal. Mr. Zhang's family was terrified after hearing this and felt fortunate for his survival.

Dr. Wang continued to explain that severe *Plasmodium falciparum* malaria often causes kidney injury and even renal failure in adult patients. The pathogenesis of renal failure is rather complex. When malaria patients develop intravascular hemolysis, large amounts of hemoglobin and malaria pigments may be present in their urine. This condition can occasionally manifest as extremely dark urine after multiple

2.3 特殊类型疟疾的临床症状有哪些？

小提示

> 特殊临床症状主要由个体因素导致。

王医生进一步解释说，老张出现的意识模糊和说胡话是脑型疟的表现。脑型疟是一种表现为意识受损、谵妄和癫痫发作的脑病。患者可能逐渐发病，也可能在惊厥后突然发作。严重程度取决于寄生虫致病力、宿主免疫应答，以及症状发作与启用治疗的时间间隔等诸多因素。在成人中，相比居住在非洲疟疾流行区的当地居民，近期去非洲的人员由于没有免疫力更常出现脑型疟，但当地人的脑型疟更多见于儿童。脑型疟非常危险，能快速导致昏迷甚至死亡，因此出现脑型疟征象后应迅速评估和处理，若不治疗，脑型疟几乎都会致命。老张一家听了后不由惊出一身汗，感叹老张命大。

王医生继续解释说，重症恶性疟的成人患者还常出现肾损伤，乃至肾衰竭。肾衰竭的发病机制非常复杂。当疟疾患者出现血管内溶血时，尿液中可能出现大量血红蛋白和疟色素。此情况偶尔可表现为多次恶性疟发作后的极深色尿液，临床上称为黑尿热，此时患者死亡率很高。疟疾患者常见因溶血所致轻度黄疸，而恶性疟感染可能发生重度黄疸，其原因是溶血、肝细胞损伤及胆汁淤积，成人中的发生率高于儿童。若肝功能障碍叠加肾损伤及其他器官功能障碍，则属于危重病例，救治的成功率会明显下降。

老张担心自己的疟疾会不会复发，王医生回答说：疟疾复发的原因有两种情况，均表现为病情消退后疾病再发。再燃是指由于治疗和宿主免疫应答不彻底，没有彻底清除血液内的疟原虫，残留在血流中的疟原虫重新繁殖增多所致。复发是指肝细胞中的一种迟发型原虫又重新释放进入外周血液，引起新一次原虫血症。再燃最常发生在数日或数周内；复发常发生在数周或数

Plasmodium falciparum malaria attacks, clinically known as "blackwater fever", with an extremely high mortality rate. Malaria patients often exhibit mild jaundice due to hemolysis, while severe jaundice can occur in falciparum malaria infections, primarily due to hemolysis, liver cell damage, and cholestasis. This incidence is more common in adults than children. If liver dysfunction is combined with kidney injury and other organ dysfunction, it indicates a critical case with a significantly lowered success rate of treatment.

Mr. Zhang was concerned about whether his malaria would recur. Dr. Wang answered that malaria recurrence is mainly due to relapse or reinfection, both of which manifest as disease recurrence after the disease subsides. Relapse refers to the recurrence of malaria symptoms due to incomplete treatment and host immune response, which fails to eradicate the malaria parasites from the blood flow, allowing the remaining parasites to multiply and increase. Recurrence refers to the re-release of a delayed parasite from liver cells into the peripheral blood, causing a new episode of parasitemia. Relapse is most commonly seen within a few days or weeks, while recurrence occurs within a few weeks or months. Cases of relapse caused by *Plasmodium falciparum* are relatively common, while *Plasmodium vivax* malaria and *Plasmodium ovale* malaria often cause recurrence a few months after initial treatment. To prevent relapse, it is necessary to use anti-malaria drugs according to standard guidelines for a sufficient course, while preventing recurrence requires using anti-recurrence drugs such as primaquine for radical cure.

2.4   Case 3   Can *Plasmodium Falciparum* Malaria be Fatal?

After Dr. Wang's explanation, Mr. Zhang was still unclear and asked, "If specific drugs are available for malaria, then shouldn't people be fine if they go to the hospital? Why do people still die from malaria?" Dr. Wang raised his glasses and shared a heartbreaking story of his own experience.

Twenty-six-year-old Mr. Li was an interpreter who had been working in an African country since graduating from university. After three years of interpreting work, he returned to China safely. However, just ten days after his return, he developed chills, shivers, and high fever. The next day, he experienced nausea, vomiting, and headaches. His family urgently sent him to a local hospital for

月内。恶性疟原虫引起的再燃较为常见，而间日疟和卵形疟常在初次发作治愈后数月引起复发。为预防再燃，需要规范足疗程使用抗疟药，而预防复发则需要使用伯氨喹等抗复发药物进行根治。

2.4 案例3 恶性疟能致人死亡吗?

老张听完王医生的解答，还是有些不太明白，问道："疟疾既然有特效药，那到了医院应该就不会有事了吧? 怎么还是会有人死于疟疾呢?"王医生抬了抬眼镜，说起了曾经亲身经历的一个令人悲伤的故事。

26岁的小李是一名翻译，大学毕业后就一直在非洲的一个国家做翻译。他一干就是3年，一直到回国都平安无事。没想到回国后10天，他就出现了畏寒、寒战和高热症状。第二天他还出现了恶心、呕吐、头痛等症状。家里人急着把他送到当地医院住院治疗，当地医院为了排除中枢神经系统感染，还给他做了很多检查，却一无所获，就按照上呼吸道感染给他用抗生素治疗了3天，却发现非但没有好转，还逐步加重。家里人只能把他送到王医生所在的医院急诊部，正待要收治入院时，小李的症状又加重了，陷入了昏迷。等到入院一查，发现小李的血小板明显减少，只有正常人的十分之一左右，同时肝肾功能都明显出了问题。当王医生从家属那里得知小李是从非洲回国没有多久后，立即送血涂片到检验科做了镜检。检验科的顾老师立马在镜下发现了问题，在显微镜下发现了大量的恶性疟原虫，不但有环状体还有配子体，红细胞的感染率超过了20‰。得知这种情况后，王医生立即开始给小李进行青蒿素抗原虫治疗，甚至还进行了血液净化治疗。但是，小李的治疗效果却不尽人意，病情急剧加重，再也没有醒过来，最终不治身亡。

老张听完王医生讲的故事，不由倒吸一口凉气，同时感叹自己的运气好。王医生说，疟疾确实有特效药，但必须在发病后尽早使用，如果恶性疟到了后期，已经发生多个脏器衰竭，那很可能再有特效药也回天乏术了。老张当时真的就是在鬼门关走了一遭，幸好家属及时把他送到了王医生所在的医院，对于

inpatient treatment. The local hospital performed numerous examinations to rule out central nervous system infection but found nothing. Mr. Li was then treated with antibiotics for three days for suspected upper respiratory infection. However, his condition did not improve but gradually worsened. His family had no choice but to send him to Dr. Wang's emergency department. Just as the doctor was about to admit him, Mr. Li's condition abruptly worsened, and he became unconscious. Upon admission, it was discovered that Mr. Li's platelet count had significantly decreased, only about one-tenth of the normal level, and simultaneously, there were problems with his liver and kidney function. When Dr. Wang learned from his family that Mr. Li had recently returned from Africa, he immediately sent a blood smear for microscopic examination. Dr. Gu of the laboratory immediately found the problem under the microscope. The examination revealed a large number of *Plasmodium falciparum*, not only ring bodies but also gametocytes, with an infection rate of over 20% in erythrocytes. In response to this situation, Dr. Wang immediately began treating Mr. Li with artemisinin-based anti-malaria therapy and even provided blood purification treatment. However, Mr. Li's treatment outcome was unsatisfactory, and his condition progressively worsened. He never regained consciousness and ultimately died.

Upon hearing the story, Mr. Zhang couldn't help but take a deep breath, and also felt grateful for his luckiness. Dr. Wang stated that specific drugs are indeed available for malaria, but they must be taken as early as possible after the onset of the disease; if malaria progresses to its severe form, with multiple organ failures having occurred, even the most potent specific drugs would likely be ineffective. At that time, Mr. Zhang was truly on the brink of death, but thankfully his family rushed to send him to the hospital where Dr. Wang was working. The treatment of *Plasmodium falciparum* malaria should have been undertaken without delay. If treated half a day earlier, it may lead to complete recovery, while a delay of half a day could result in rapid deterioration. Therefore, perhaps it is more attributable to Mr. Zhang's family who made decisive decision to seek medical treatment, which was the crucial factor, and reminded the doctor of Mr. Zhang's travel history to Africa.

恶性疟的治疗就应该争分夺秒，早半天治疗或许就能够痊愈，晚半天治疗病情可能就急速恶化，因此或许更应该要感谢的是老张的家属，当时果断地决定送医治疗才是关键中的关键，并提醒了医生患者曾去过非洲的旅行史。

2.5 如何通过临床症状判别重症疟疾？

小提示

（1）重症疟疾的临床症状包括意识改变、呼吸窘迫、循环衰竭、血红蛋白尿（黑尿热）等。

（2）查体可能发现苍白、瘀点、黄疸、肝肿大和脾肿大等。

（3）临床检验可以发现代谢性酸中毒、肝肾功能衰竭、肝功能衰竭、凝血障碍、重度贫血和低血糖等。

王医生继续说道，对于老张，之前其实也已经进展为重症疟疾，重症疟疾的临床表现包括意识改变（伴或不伴有癫痫发作）、呼吸窘迫或急性呼吸窘迫综合征，循环衰竭、代谢性酸中毒、肾衰竭、血红蛋白尿（黑尿热）、肝功能衰竭、凝血障碍（伴或不伴有弥散性血管内凝血）、重度贫血或大量血管内溶血、低血糖等。虽然上述症状往往会一同出现，但由于都会威胁生命，因此只要有一条就可以诊断为重症疟疾。重症疟疾的临床表现各种各样，任何一种都是人体器官明显受损的表现，都有可能威胁生命，因此都需要引起临床医生的高度重视。

虽然绝大多数重症疟疾为恶性疟原虫所致，但间日疟原虫也会引起重症疟疾。重症疟疾的极高危人群包括：以往没有感染过疟疾的无免疫力个体、免疫功能受损患者，儿童及孕妇。血中的疟原虫密度越高，患者病情通常也越重。一些重症或治疗不当的患者在初次就诊时，原虫血症水平可能较低，但之后会逐渐升高。疟疾患者一旦出现了重症疟疾的这些并发症时，说明病情危重有生命危险，这时临床医生应迅速开展全面评估并立即治疗。

2.5　How to Distinguish Severe Malaria through Clinical Symptoms?

Tips

(1) Clinical symptoms of severe malaria include altered mental states, respiratory distress, circulatory failure, hemoglobinuria (blackwater fever) etc.

(2) Physical examination may reveal pallor, petechiae, jaundice, hepatomegaly, and spleen enlargement, etc.

(3) Clinical tests can show metabolic acidosis, hepatic and renal failure, hepatic failure, blood coagulation disorders, severe anemia, and hypoglycemia, etc.

Dr. Wang continued, "In fact, Mr. Zhang's condition had also progressed to severe malaria." Clinical Symptoms of severe malaria include altered mental states (with or without epileptic seizures), respiratory distress or acute respiratory distress syndrome, circulatory failure, metabolic acidosis, renal failure, hemoglobinuria (blackwater fever), hepatic failure, blood coagulation disorders with or without disseminated intravascular coagulation, severe anemia or massive intravascular hemolysis, and hypoglycemia. Although these symptoms often occur together, they can threaten life individually. Therefore, any one of them can be diagnosed as severe malaria. It thus follows that the clinical manifestations of severe malaria are diverse and any one of them represents significant organ damage in the human body, posing a potential threat to life. Therefore, they should all elicit high attention from clinical doctors.

Although is the primary cause of most severe cases of *Plasmodium falciparum infection*, *Plasmodium vivax* can also induce it. The extremely high-risk population of severe malaria includes individuals with no prior malaria infection and compromised immunity, as well as children and pregnant women. Generally, the higher the density of malaria parasites in the blood, the more severe the patient's condition. Some patients with severe malaria or improper treatment may have a lower level of parasitemia at the initial visit but gradually experience an increase. Once these complications of severe malaria appear, it indicates a critical condition and life-threatening situation. Clinical doctors should promptly conduct a comprehensive assessment and immediate treatment.

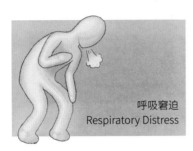
呼吸窘迫
Respiratory Distress

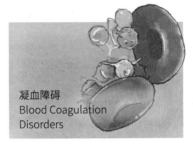
凝血障碍
Blood Coagulation
Disorders

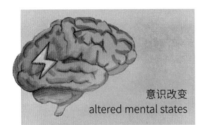
意识改变
altered mental states

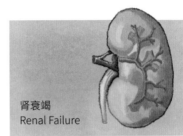
肾衰竭
Renal Failure

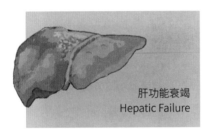
肝功能衰竭
Hepatic Failure

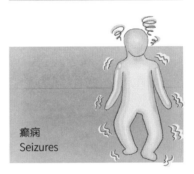
癫痫
Seizures

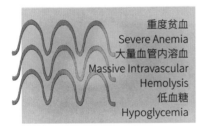
重度贫血
Severe Anemia
大量血管内溶血
Massive Intravascular
Hemolysis
低血糖
Hypoglycemia

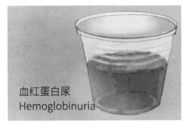
血红蛋白尿
Hemoglobinuria

图 2-3 重症疟疾的临床症状
Figure 2-3 Clinical Symptoms of Severe Malaria

③ Risk Populations and Prevention

3.1   Who are the High-Risk Groups for Malaria?

Malaria parasites could infect anyone, regardless of your race, gender, age, or occupation. However, under the same environment, children who have weaker immunity and pregnant women are more Drone to severe symptoms after infection (data shows that the rates of incidence and malaria parasites in children are significantly higher than those in adults). There are also populations from non-endemic regions having no immunity against malaria parasites. Who enter malaria-endemic regions to seek refuge from natural disasters or war, or simply find jobs, making them particularly vulnerable to malaria parasites and infection.

Conversely, humans possess genetic traits that result in varying degrees of our reactivity to malaria parasite infections and different susceptibilities to specific species of malaria parasites. Individuals with special immune diseases, such as Duffy-negative phenotype, sickle cell anemia, and thalassemia, exhibit lower susceptibility to *Plasmodium falciparum* or experience milder symptoms following infection.

People of different races, genders, ages, and occupations are susceptible to all four species of malaria parasites. In the early stages of a malaria outbreak, given that the population lacks immunity, when the epidemic continues, the incidence and the parasite rates in children would significantly be higher than those in adults, pregnant women who have lower immunity and are more susceptible to malaria. Furthermore, individuals with low immunity to malaria are easily infected when entering highly endemic regions for reasons such as seeking work or seeking refuge, etc. Due to differences in lifestyle, clothing, and working conditions, as well as exposure to mosquito bites, the malaria infection rate sometimes varies among people of different genders and occupations.

Overall, infants, children under 5, pregnant women, HIV/AIDS cases, immune-deficient migrants, migrant population, and travelers have poor or no immunity to malaria are the most susceptible groups to infection. Moreover, their symptoms are often more severe and could even lead to death.

③ 危险人群与预防

3.1　哪些人是疟疾高风险人群？

疟原虫不挑人，不论你是何种族、是男是女、是幼是老、从事何种职业，几乎"通吃"所有人群。不过，在同等环境下，免疫力低的儿童、妊娠期妇女感染后症状更重（数据显示，儿童的发病率和原虫率都显著高于成人）。还有一些非流行区的人群，也是对疟原虫无任何免疫力的人，他们为了逃避自然灾害、战乱或仅仅为了找工作进入了疟疾流行区，就特别容易被疟原虫盯上，感染的风险很高。

反过来，我们人类也有一些遗传特质，使得我们对疟原虫感染的反应程度有所不同，对特定种类的疟原虫的易感情况也不一样的。有些患有特殊免疫疾病的人群，如 Duffy 抗原血型阴性、镰刀红细胞症患者、地中海贫血患者对间日疟原虫不易感或感染后症状比较轻微。

不同种族、性别、年龄和职业的人对 4 种疟原虫都是易感的。在疟疾暴发初期，人群缺乏免疫力，随着流行的持续，儿童的发病率和原虫率都显著高于成人；妊娠期妇女免疫力较低，易感染疟疾。此外，当对疟疾具有低免疫力的人群进入疟疾高度传播地区找工作或者避难时也很容易感染疟疾；不同性别和职业的人由于生活习惯、衣着、劳动条件等不同或是暴露给蚊媒叮咬的机会不同，疟疾感染率有时也不一样。

总体来说，婴儿、小于 5 岁的儿童、孕妇和 HIV/AIDS 病例、无免疫力的移民、流动人口以及旅行者对疟疾的免疫力较差或毫无免疫力，最易感染疟疾，且感染后症状往往较重，甚至死亡。

📖 Extended Reading

Negative in Duffy antigen blood group (3CA). The Duffy blood group consists of two main antigens: Fya and Fyb. Based on the presence of these antigens on erythrocytes, the Duffy blood group can be divided into Fy (a⁺b⁻), Fy (a⁻b⁺), Fy (a⁺b⁺), and Fy (a⁻b⁻). Research has found that the Fy antigen in the Duffy blood group is a receptor for *Plasmodium vivax* binding to erythrocytes. Individuals with negative Fy (a⁻b⁻) in Duffy blood group have no such receptor on the erythrocyte membrane, so *Plasmodium vivax* cannot invade erythrocytes, making them less susceptible to *Plasmodium falciparum*.

Sickle Cell Disease(SCD): It is a genetic blood disease that under ordinary microscopy shows abnormal crescent-shaped (or sickle-like) erythrocytes. This is mainly due to a single base substitution in the DNA sequence of the gene encoding the β-chain of hemoglobin (the protein carrying oxygen in erythrocytes). Sickle cell anemia occurs when an individual inherits two copies of the sickle mutation (one from the mother and one from the father), resulting in sickle cell anemia. SCD can impair the oxygen-carrying capacity of erythrocytes, reducing the potassium ion concentration within them. Meanwhile, as sickle cell hemoglobin is not water-soluble, it hinders the phagocytosis and pinocytosis of *Plasmodium falciparum*. Under low oxygen pressure, hemoglobin can form microcrystals that puncture the malaria parasite's surface membrane, thus affecting its survival.

β-TDT: It is a common genetic disorder caused by defects in the hemoglobin gene, which reduces or prevents the synthesis of one or more globin peptide chains in hemoglobin. This results in abnormal hemoglobin quantity and quality, making erythrocytes more susceptible to destruction by the liver and spleen, shortening their lifespan, and leading to anemia and even developmental abnormalities. It also affects the growth and development of malaria parasites, thereby preventing infection.

How can high-risk populations avoid and prevent malaria? Currently, there are several measures:

(1) Collective prophylactic medication: A protective measure for high-risk populations during malaria transmission seasons. It is often implemented in the following situations—to curb the spread and rapidly reduce incidence in severe endemic or outbreak regions; to prevent the occurrence of new outbreaks in post malaria elimination regions where imported secondary cases appear; to conduct collective prophylactic medication, to prevent outbreaks in regions with a large number of high-malaria-risk population, such as mines and large-scale construction sites.

> **拓展阅读**
>
> Duffy 抗原血型阴性（SCA）：Duffy 血型主要有两种抗原：Fya 和 Fyb，以红细胞上携带这两种抗原的情况来看，Duffy 血型可以分为 Fy（a⁺b⁻）、Fy（a⁻b⁺）、Fy（a⁺b⁺）和 Fy（a⁻b⁻）。经研究发现，Duffy 血型 Fy 抗原是间日疟原虫结合红细胞的受体，Duffy 血型阴性 Fy（a⁻b⁻）的个体红细胞膜上无此受体，因而间日疟原虫不能入侵红细胞，使其不易感。
>
> 镰刀型红细胞贫血（SCD）：是一种具有遗传性的血液病，普通显微镜下显示其红细胞呈异常新月状（或镰刀样），主要是由于编码血红蛋白（红细胞内携带氧的蛋白）β 链的基因 DNA 序列上的单个碱基发生了置换。当个体遗传了 2 个拷贝镰状突变（1 个源自母亲，另 1 个源自父亲）时，就会发生镰状细胞性贫血。镰刀型红细胞贫血可削弱红细胞的携氧能力，使红细胞内钾离子浓度降低，与此同时，由于镰状细胞血红蛋白不溶于水，会阻碍恶性疟原虫的吞噬和胞饮作用，在氧压低时，血红蛋白可形成微晶，刺破疟原虫表面膜，从而影响其存活。
>
> β-地中海贫血（TDT）：是常见的基因缺陷性疾病，主要是由于珠蛋白基因的缺陷使血红蛋白中的珠蛋白肽链有一种或几种合成减少或不能合成，血红蛋白数量和质量异常，使红细胞容易被人体的肝脾等破坏，寿命缩短，导致贫血甚至发育异常，对疟原虫生长发育产生影响，从而阻碍了疟原虫的感染。

那高危人群应如何避免和预防疟疾呢？目前主要有以下措施。

（1）集体预防服药：指在疟疾传播季节，针对高危人群的一种保护措施。常在下列情况时实施——在严重流行或暴发地区，遏制流行的扩散蔓延及迅速降低发病率；在疟疾已被消除的地区，用于出现输入继发病例的疫点，以防止发生新的流行；在有大量高疟区人群进入的矿山、大型建筑工地等，开展集体预防服药以防止疟疾暴发。

（2）个人预防服药：非疟区无免疫力的人群进入疟区时，应于传播季节定期服用抗疟药物，以预防感染。特别是到高疟区的人员，更应注意加强个人预防。疟疾流行区夜晚室外作业与野外住宿者等高危人群，在传播季节也

(2) Personal prophylactic medication: When population without immunity to malaria enters malaria-endemic regions during the transmission season, they should take anti-malaria drugs regularly to prevent infection. Particularly for outdoor workers and campers in malaria-endemic regions during transmission season, as well as those travelling to high-risk regions, personal prevention should also be strengthened.

(3) When symptoms such as periodic chills, fever, and sweating occur, immediately go to any types of medical and disease control facilities at any levels for blood tests of malaria or other pathological examinations for timely diagnosis and symptomatic treatment.

3.2 What Methods can Prevent Malaria?

Since malaria is transmitted via mosquito bites, when infected mosquitoes bite non-infected population bite malaria patients, they can spread malaria to the healthy people. Thus, the key factor in preventing malaria is to prevent mosquito bites. To prevent mosquito bites, the followings should be taken into account.

1. Remove and control mosquito breeding sites:

Malaria relies on mosquitoes for transmission, so killing mosquitoes and preventing mosquito bites should be the top priority;

Timely clean wastewater and garbage, and kill mosquitoes and flies with residual spraying of insecticides.

(1) Improve environmental and residential hygiene: For example, fill up useless water puddles, depressions, and ditches, drain stagnant water from channels, pipes, and sewers, clear weeds, and make inverted any containers that accumulate water, such as pans and buckets, to keep the living area clean and tidy.

(2) Use insecticides for indoor residual spraying and outdoor spraying (especially in sewers): Residual spraying involves applying long-lasting insecticide solutions to indoor walls, doors, windows, ceilings, and furniture surfaces, allowing the insecticide to remain on the surfaces for a longer period and to maintain its efficacy. This method is suitable for spraying residential houses, offices, hotels, cafeterias, warehouses, air raid shelters, and toilets to kill mosquitoes, lasting 2-3 months. Indoor residual spraying of insecticides is a powerful measure to rapidly

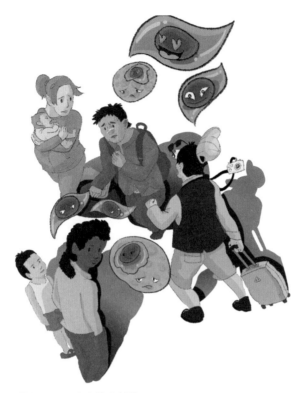

图 3-1　疟疾易感人群
Figure 3-1　Susceptible Population to Malaria

应进行预防服药，并加强个体防护。

　　（3）当出现具有周期性的发冷、发热、出汗等症状时，应立即前往各级各类医疗、疾控机构进行疟原虫血检或以其他检验方法及时确诊并对症治疗。

3.2　哪些手段可以预防疟疾？

　　由于疟疾是被蚊虫叮咬而传染的，蚊虫叮咬疟疾患者后，再叮咬健康人时就会把疟疾传到健康人的身上，使人发病。因此，预防疟疾的关键是防止蚊虫叮咬。防止蚊虫叮咬，可以从以下几个方面考虑。

reduce malaria transmission.

2. Reduce human-mosquito contact:

Insecticide-treated net has a long-lasting effect, and is simple, safe, and easy to use;

Improving living conditions is the key. The intactness of window screens and door screens should be ensured;

The environment should be equipped with mosquito-repellent zones, insecticides to kill mosquitoes and insects should be applied regularly;

Avoid going out during dawn and dusk, Stay away from wetlands and grasslands;

Wear long-sleeved cloths and trousers when going outside, and apply mosquito repellent to exposed skin.

(1) Utilizing insecticide-treated nets: Insecticide-treated nets such as pyrethroid are highly efficient. They have long-lasting efficacy and repellent properties and may reduce blood feeding rates and malaria incidence. Their usage is straightforward which can be easily used by the mass. It is also low-cost and safe for humans and animals, hence serves as a crucial measures to rapidly reduce malaria incidence. These insecticide-treated nets as a physical barrier can minimize contact between mosquitoes and humans, provide insecticidal effects.

(2) Improving living conditions and habits: Install window screens and door screens, close doors and windows, avoid outdoor sleeping, spray insecticides or burn mosquito coils in bedrooms, and use nets or long-lasting nets while sleeping.

(3) Crop protection: Plant drought-resistant crops around villages and between rice paddies and maintain an appropriate width as a mosquito-repellent zone.

(4) Minimizing outdoor activities during mosquito activity peaks (dawn and dusk): If outdoor activities is unavoidable, wear long-sleeved shirts and long pants, and apply external mosquito repellents to exposed skin to prevent mosquito bites.

3. Physical mosquito repellent

The importance of physical mosquito repellent cannot be overlooked, with mosquito trap lamps and electric mosquito swatters being essential tools.

The mosquito trap lamp attracts mosquitoes and midges, while the high-voltage grid efficiently kills them.

This utilizes the phototaxis and sensitivity to specific wavelengths of mosquitoes. A mosquito trap lamp with a power of 8W and a wavelength of 253.7nm is recommended. The mosquito trap lamp should ideally be placed in a

1. 清除和控制蚊虫滋生地

疟疾依靠蚊子传，灭蚊防蚊要当先；

污水垃圾及时清，滞留喷洒灭蚊蝇。

（1）搞好环境和居室卫生：如填平无用的水坑、洼地、水沟，将无用积水排出沟渠、管道、阴沟，清除杂草，将盆、桶等各种能够积水的器皿倒置等，保持居住区周围干净整洁。

（2）使用杀虫剂进行室内滞留喷洒和室外（尤其是下水道）喷洒：滞留喷洒是把持效期长的杀虫剂药液喷洒在室内的墙壁、门窗、天花板和家具等表面上，使药剂滞留在上述物体表面，维持较长时期的药效。适用于喷洒住房、办公室、宾馆、食堂、仓库、防空洞和厕所等场所，以杀灭蚊虫，持续时间一般为 2～3 个月。室内滞留喷洒是迅速减少疟疾传播的有力措施。

2. 减少人蚊接触

药浸蚊帐持效长，简单安全易使用；

改善条件是关键，保持完好门纱窗；

环境要设防蚊带，定期施药杀蚊虫；

黎明黄昏少外出，避开湿地和草丛；

外出长袖和长裤，暴露皮肤驱蚊剂。

（1）使用药浸蚊帐：拟除虫菊酯等杀虫剂处理蚊帐具有高效、长特效、趋避、减少吸血率和降低疟疾发病率的作用，且使用方法简单，群众易使用，成本低，对人畜安全，是迅速降低疟疾发病率的重要措施之一。睡在药浸蚊帐里可以减少蚊虫与人体之间的接触，它提供了物理屏障，且具有杀虫效果。

（2）改善居住条件和习惯：安装纱门、纱窗，出入随手关门窗，改变室外露宿的习惯，可在卧室喷洒杀虫剂或点蚊香，睡觉时使用蚊帐或使用长效蚊帐。

hidden corner that is higher than 1m but no more than 1.8m from the ground. To maximize the lamp's effectiveness, turn off all indoor light sources, as other light sources can interfere with mosquitoes, distracting them from sensing the sources of the mosquito trap lamp which significantly reduces its mosquito-attracting effect. We can also use an electric mosquito swatter, which attracts mosquitoes with its UV light, leading them to contact the mesh, then die instantly from the high-voltage electric shock, to prevent mosquito bites.

4. Chemical mosquito repellent

Always having mosquito repellent liquid on hand and spraying it promptly;

Using electric mosquito repellent incense to guarantee a peaceful night's sleep.

(1) Mosquito coil is the oldest natural method of mosquito repellent, herbal mosquito repellent stick was invented back to Southern Song Dynasty. The active pyrethrin of modern mosquito coils is the main ingredient, with a repellent and killing effect on mosquitoes. When a mosquito coil is lit, the pyrethrin in it evaporates into the indoor air, paralyzing the mosquito's nerves, causing them to either die or flee, thus repelling and killing mosquitoes. Pyrethrin is metabolically excreted and poses little harm to humans. However, low-quality mosquito coils contain not only pyrethrin but also toxic substances such as BHC and realgar powder, which can be harmful to humans and even cause cancer. Therefore, it's best to use mosquito coils outdoors, such as around the house, at the entrance, or in well-ventilated regions. Lighting a mosquito coil an hour before sunset provides the best repellent effect.

(2) The repellent effect of electric mosquito repellent mats is also excellent, generally lasting 6 to 8 hours. They absorb pyrethrin into a patch and heat it up for evaporation. Adding a few drops of wind medicated oil can enhance the effect. Liquid mosquito repellent mats, following the capillary principle, continuously release insecticide substances, making them a convenient option. A bottle of mosquito repellent liquid used for 8 hours a day can last 30 days, avoiding the hassling of daily replacement of electric mosquito repellent mats. However, both electric mosquito repellent mats and mosquito repellent liquid contain harmful organic compounds. If used in a closed room, they may cause adverse reactions. Therefore, guarantee good air circulation when using electric mosquito repellent. The optimal usage time is half an hour before going to bed.

(3) Mosquito repellent liquid, also known as mosquito repellent, is mainly used

（3）作物防护：在村庄周围和稻田之间种植旱作物并保持适宜宽度作为防蚊带。

（4）尽量避免在蚊虫活动高峰期（黄昏和夜晚）到户外活动：如必须在户外工作，可穿长袖衣和长裤，皮肤暴露处可涂抹外驱蚊剂，防蚊叮咬。

3. 物理驱蚊

物理驱蚊亦重要，蚊灯蚊拍少不了。

诱蚊灯管引蚊虫，电网杀蚊效率高。

可以利用蚊虫的趋光性及对特殊波长的敏感性，选择功率为 8W、波长为 253.7nm 的诱蚊灯。诱蚊灯最好放置在高于 1m，且离地面不超过 180cm 的隐蔽角落。使用诱蚊灯时，室内光源最好全部关闭，因为蚊虫会被其他光源干扰，无法感受到诱蚊灯的光源，诱蚊效果也将大减。我们也可以使用电蚊拍，利用电蚊拍紫外光对蚊子的吸引力，以灯管诱捕蚊虫接触网面，并用高压电击网丝，瞬间使蚊子烧焦，从而防止蚊虫叮咬。

4. 化学驱蚊

常备防蚊液，及时喷一喷；

电热蚊香液，安睡一整夜。

（1）蚊香是最古老的天然药物驱蚊办法。早在南宋时期便出现过中药制成的驱蚊香棒。现代蚊香中的有效成分主要是除虫菊酯等杀虫药，它有驱杀蚊虫的作用。蚊香点燃后，蚊香里的除虫菊酯随着烟雾挥发出来，播散于室内的空气中，使蚊子的神经麻痹，于是蚊子或坠地丧命，或四散逃跑，从而起到驱灭蚊虫的作用。除虫菊酯可以通过代谢排出体外，对人没有多大害处。但是某些低劣的蚊香，除含有除虫菊酯之外，还含有六六六粉、雄黄粉等，这些物质对人体有毒性甚至致癌作用。因此，蚊香最好还是放在户外使用，比如房子周围、门口或空气流通的地方。傍晚天黑前点燃蚊香，驱蚊效果最佳。

by people who spend time outdoors or work in the wild. The main ingredient of mosquito repellent liquid is DEET. When applied correctly, it can effectively prevent mosquito bites within a certain period of time. The drug may directly act on the mosquito's tactile organs and chemical sensors, driving away mosquitoes. When children use mosquito repellent liquid, special care should be taken, and it's best to use liquids with a DEET concentration of less than 10%. Infants are prone to licking the liquid and poisoning themselves, so it's better not to use it. When applying mosquito repellent liquid, avoid spraying it directly on wounds or skin with rashes. You can first spray it on your hands and then apply it to exposed body parts accordingly, which can be less convenient.

(4) Mosquito-killing aerosols contain an active ingredient prallethrin, which is effective against mosquitoes that typically hide in dark, damp places namely stairwells, under sinks, gutters, bathrooms, cabinets, and under the tables. By setting up an "artificial trap" made of old boxes or barrels filled with towels to create a dark, damp environment, mosquitoes will be attracted to rest inside. Hence, spraying insecticide inside the trap will effectively eradicate mosquitoes.

(5) Mosquito-killing window screen coating utilizes the phototropism of mosquitoes and the slow-release principle of medicines. A protective film is formed by applying the mosquito-killing coating on window screens. After 30 seconds of contact, mosquitoes and flies will die within 2 hours to several days. The active ingredients are generally permethrin and cypermethrin, etc. However, do not clean the window screens with alkaline solvents. This coating is durable, resistant to sunlight and washing, and may last several months to half a year.

（2）电蚊香片的驱蚊效果也不错，一般可维持 6～8 个小时。电蚊香的驱蚊原理是将除虫菊等吸入蚊香片中，加热后蒸发，滴上数滴风油精效果更好。液体电蚊香是利用毛细管原理，持续加热释放杀虫剂物质，使用最为方便。按每天使用 8 小时计算，一瓶蚊香液可连续使用 30 天，免除了每天更换电蚊香片的麻烦。但无论是电蚊香片还是液体电蚊香，都含有对人体有害的有机化合物。如在密闭房间内使用，可能会产生不良反应。因此，使用电蚊香时应保持空气流通。电蚊香的最佳使用时间是睡前半小时。

（3）防蚊液，又称驱蚊剂，主要用于外出或野外作业人员。防蚊液的主要成分是避蚊胺。涂抹质量合格的防蚊液可以在一定时间内有效防止蚊虫叮咬。其原理是药物直接作用于蚊虫的触觉器官及化学感受器，从而驱赶蚊虫。孩子使用防蚊液应特别留心，最好使用避蚊胺浓度小于 10% 的防蚊液。婴儿涂抹容易误舔食中毒，最好不用。喷涂防蚊液时，避免直接洒在伤口或是起红疹的皮肤上。可先喷在手上，然后在身体裸露部位皮肤上一一涂抹，使用起来有点麻烦。

（4）杀蚊气雾剂是一种杀虫剂，其主要化学成分是一种叫作炔丙菊酯的物质。蚊子多半喜欢躲在阴暗潮湿的地方，白天针对楼梯间、水槽下、阴沟、浴厕、橱柜、桌脚下等喷洒。利用旧箱子或桶子，放些抹布在里面，布置成一个阴暗潮湿的"人工陷阱"，白天蚊子飞进去歇息，往里头喷几下杀虫剂，就可以轻松灭蚊。

（5）灭蚊窗纱涂剂是利用蚊虫的向光性和药物的缓释原理，将灭蚊窗纱涂剂涂抹在纱窗上，形成一层保护膜，蚊蝇接触 30 秒后，会在 2 小时至数日内死亡。有效灭蚊成分一般为氯菊酯（扑灭司林）、氯氢菊酯等。使用时，勿用碱性溶剂清洗窗纱。其优点是耐日晒耐水洗，有效时间长达数月至半年。

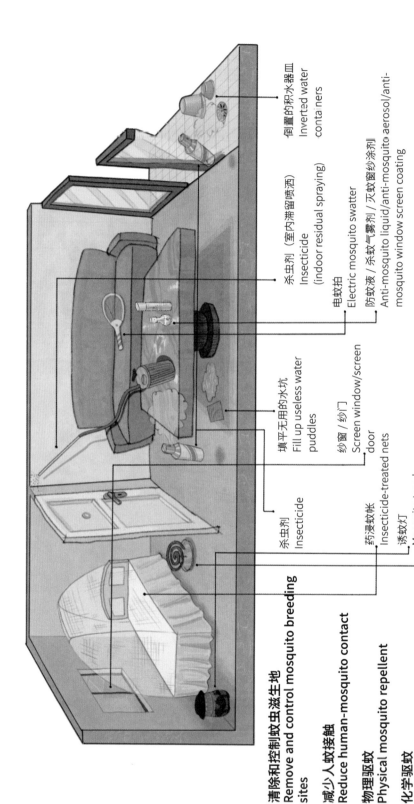

倒置的积水器皿
Inverted water conta ners

杀虫剂（室内滞留喷洒）
Insecticide
(indoor residual spraying)

电蚊拍
Electric mosquito swatter

防蚊液／杀蚊气雾剂／灭蚊窗纱涂剂
Anti-mosquito liquid/anti-mosquito aerosol/anti-mosquito window screen coating

填平无用的水坑
Fill up useless water puddles

纱窗（纱）门
Screen window/screen door

杀虫剂
Insecticide

药浸蚊帐
Insecticide-treated nets

诱蚊灯
Mosquito trap lamp

蚊香／电蚊香
Mosquito repellent/Electric mosquito repellent

清除和控制蚊虫滋生地
Remove and control mosquito breeding sites

减少人蚊接触
Reduce human-mosquito contact

物理驱蚊
Physical mosquito repellent

化学驱蚊
Chemical mosquito repellent

图 3-2 防蚊小妙招
Figure 3-2 Tips for Preventing Mosquito Bites

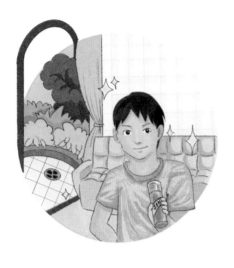
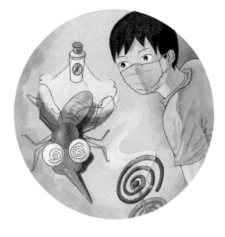

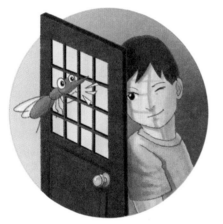
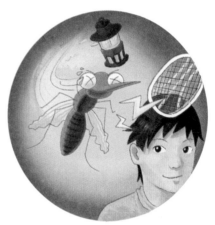
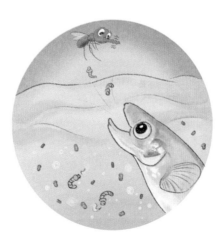

Tips

Long-term use of the same chemical mosquito repellent can lead to resistance in mosquitoes, so it is recommended to alternate different mosquito repellent methods and products to achieve better results.

5. Biological mosquito killing

Biological mosquito killing is long-lasting and can be achieved by keeping certain animals;

Raising mosquito-eating fish in pool water and using bacillus to kill larvae is an environmentally friendly method.

Predatory animals can also be used to kill mosquitoes. For example, common carp and mosquito-eating fish can prevent the breeding of mosquito larvae in paddy fields, ponds, and reservoirs. *Bacillus thuringiensis* and *Bacillus sphaericus* are used for biological killing of mosquito larvae.

In summary, there are various ways to prevent mosquito bites, and the safest and most effective methods are keeping the living environment clean, improving living conditions, and adopting physical repellents.

3.3 Case 4 Is Biological Killing of Mosquito Larvae Effective?

Providing long-lasting insecticide-treated nets and using indoor residual spraying of insecticides in the homes of high-risk population are specific measures in the control of malaria transmission included in the key interventions for malaria prevention and control programmes recommended by the WHO. These two measures have been recognized worldwide for their achievements in controlling malaria transmission, but they also face issues such as inconvenience of and resistance to using nets, as well as environmental impact and the emergence of insecticides resistant mosquitoes. Additionally, there are multiple species of mosquitoes, with distinct habits, diets, and preferences that transmit malaria. Some prefer to feed on human blood, while others prefer cattle blood. Some move to the bedroom after dinner, while others return to the water's edge after a hearty meal... Not all mosquitoes can be easily controlled by human strategies. So, is there a method to control all mosquitoes? To find it out, we need to look into commonalities among mosquitoes. What do mosquitoes have in common? Yes, their larvae, called

　　长时间使用同种化学驱蚊剂，蚊虫会对其产生一定的抗药性，因此我们应该轮流使用不同的驱蚊方法及产品，才能获得更好的驱蚊效果。

　　5. 生物灭蚊

　　生物灭蚊持效长，养养动物可实现；

　　池水放养柳条鱼，杆菌灭幼真环保。

　　捕食性动物也可用于灭蚊。例如，家鱼、柳条鱼可防止稻田、池塘和水库中的媒介按蚊幼虫的繁殖。苏云金杆菌、球形芽孢杆菌可用于生物灭蚊蚴。

　　总之，防蚊方法多种多样，最安全、有效的当属保持环境卫生、改善居住条件和采用物理驱蚊方法。

3.3　案例 4　生物灭蚊蚴有效吗？

　　为高风险人群提供长效药浸蚊帐和对其家庭环境使用杀虫剂室内滞留喷洒，是世界卫生组织制定的疟疾防治关键干预措施中涉及媒介控制中的具体措施。此两种措施在控制疟疾传播方面所取得的成就已经得到全世界的认可，却也面临不少问题：如嫌蚊帐太闷而不用蚊帐、对环境的影响，以及耐药性蚊子的出现。另外，传播疟疾的蚊子有很多种，不同蚊子的饮食习惯、性格、爱好不尽相同，有的喜欢吸人血，有的喜欢吸牛血，有的吃完晚饭直接住在卧室，还有的饱餐后回到水边……可不是所有的蚊子都会按照人们的计谋乖乖就范的。那么有没有一种方法能对付所有的蚊子呢？那我们就要"找共同点"，蚊子有什么共同点呢？对啦，蚊子的幼虫——子孓都住在水里，如果能有一种方法杀灭子孓，岂不是将蚊子统统扼杀在摇篮中了？

　　生物灭蚊蚴就是这样一种方法。1964 年，凯伦和迈尔斯发现球形芽孢杆

wigglers, all live in water. If there were a way to kill the wigglers, wouldn't it effectively kill mosquitoes in the early phases?

Biological control targeting on mosquito larvae is a method of this sort. In 1964, Kellen and Meyers discovered that *Bacillus sphaericus* (Bs) could achieve the purpose of malaria prevention and control by killing mosquito larva in water. Bs is an insect pathogen, and its toxic effect on mosquitoes is primarily due to the toxins produced during its growth, which increase the permeability of epithelial cell membranes of sensitive mosquitoes, resulting in cell swelling, and ultimately the death of mosquito larva. Moreover, the spores of Bs re-circulate within the dead mosquito larvae and under certain environmental conditions, resulting in a long-lasting period of application in the wild. Most importantly, Bs is essentially a bacterium and leaves no impact on the environment. Biological control on mosquito larvae has achieved remarkable results in urban mosquito control. Starting form the 1980s, the application of *Bacillus thuringiensis* and Bs to kill mosquito larva in the upper reaches of the Rhine River in Germany continued for over a decade, with the population density of mosquitoes decreasing by 90% each year, becoming a successful model of biological control on mosquito larvae. However, for some reasons, the Bs method has been mostly limited to experimental and applied research in the control of malaria vectors, with very few large-scale field applications. In the early 21st century, Henan Province also implemented biological control on mosquito larvae in response to the rising malaria outbreaks in the Huanghuai Plain region, achieving positive results alongside conventional vector control measures for controlling malaria transmission.

Since 2003, the malaria endemic in Yongcheng City, Henan Province, located in the heart of the Huanghuai Plain, has gradually rebounded. The number of malaria cases has increased exponentially for three consecutive years, reaching 36 outbreak points in four townships by 2006. To curb the rapidly rising endemic, Yongcheng City initiated biological killing of mosquito larvae in villages with a high number of malaria cases. Before implementing the measures, sufficient preparations were needed, including purchasing equipment and reagents, training personnel, and conducting extensive publicity campaigns to garner more public support, surveying various water bodies within and around the village to calculate the dosage of Bs, investigating the density of adult mosquitoes and wigglers to provide reference data for evaluating the effect of the later phases. From August to October 2007, Bs suspension was sprayed on various water bodies in the village and its surroundings

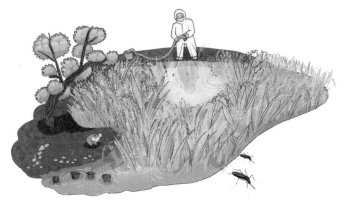

水体使用球形芽孢杆菌消灭按蚊幼虫
Killing anopheles mosquito larvae with *Bacillus sphaericus* in water bodies

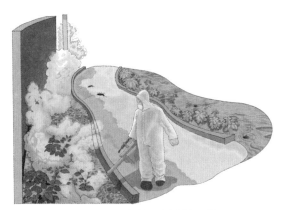

环境喷洒杀虫剂消灭蚊子
Spraying insecticides in the environment to kill mosquitoes

图 3-3　生物灭蚊蚴
Figure 3-3　Biological Killing of Mosquito Larvae

菌（*Bacillus sphaericus*，Bs）可通过杀灭水中的孑孓而达到防治疟疾的目的。Bs 是一种昆虫病原菌，杀蚊毒性主要是由于在生长过程中产生的毒素，通过增加敏感蚊虫上皮细胞膜的通透性，引起细胞膨胀，最终导致蚊子孑死亡。此外，Bs 的芽孢在死蚊幼虫体内和一定的环境下发生再循环，野外应用持续期长。最重要的是，Bs 的本质是细菌，对环境没有影响。生物灭蚊蚴措施在城市灭蚊方面取得了显著成效，20 世纪 80 年代开始，在德国的莱茵河上游连续 10 多年采用苏云金杆菌和 Bs 灭蚊蚴虫，蚊虫种群密度每年下降

every 15 days, with a dosage of 8ml Bs per square meter of water surface. After the spraying, the larvae of *Anopheles sinensis* decreased by 75.6% to 100%, adult mosquitoes decreased by 56% to 100%, and the incidence of malaria decreased by 51.3% compared to the previous year. This demonstrated that the biological killing of mosquito larvae with Bs was an effective approach in controlling malaria transmission and reducing the number of malaria cases.

Tips

1. Advantages of biological killing of mosquito larvae

(1) Biological larviciding using Bs offers a safer alternative to traditional chemical control methods. It is harmless to other insects, fish, birds, mammals, and humans at recommended doses.

(2) Biological larviciding is particularly advantageous in regions where mosquitoes have developed resistance to chemical insecticides.

(3) From a cost effectiveness perspective, the expenditure for biological larviciding is reasonable and is comparable to other mosquito-borne intervention measures.

2. Feasibility of biological killing of mosquito larvae

It is widely recognized that regions with seasonal occurrences or relatively fewer, distinctively bounded, and easily accessible larval habitats, coupled with high population densities sufficient for repeated treatment of breeding sites, may yield the most effective and cost-efficient methods for controlling mosquito larvae. Such environments are prevalent in sub-Saharan Africa. Drawing upon previous research findings, it has been noted that African malaria-transmitting *Anopheles* mosquitoes are highly sensitive to Bs and the Israeli subspecies of *Bacillus thuringiensis* (Bti). Consequently, biological killing of mosquito larvae could serve as an effective tool for malaria prevention and control in African regions.

3. Promotion of biological killing of mosquito larvae

The promotion of biological killing of mosquito larvae in African region can draw on Chinese experience and focus on the following aspects:

(1) Establish policy support for management planning of mosquito larvae sources;

(2) Conduct baseline mapping and data collection, including water body habitats and population data of larvae and adults;

(3) Provide training for local staff;

(4) Engage in widespread publicity to raise community awareness.

90%，成为生物灭蚊的成功典范。然而，不知为何，Bs 从诞生起，在控制疟疾媒介方面大多仅局限于试验和应用性研究，大规模现场应用少之又少。21世纪初，河南省在应对黄淮平原疟疾疫情回升时，除常规的传染源管理结合媒介控制措施外，开展了生物灭蚊蚴措施，取得了较好的效果。

2003 年起，位于黄淮平原腹地的河南省永城市疟疾疫情逐渐回升，疟疾发病连续 3 年呈倍数增长，到 2006 年，4 个乡镇出现 36 个疟疾暴发点。为控制疫情快速上升的势头，永城市在疟疾病例较多的村庄实施了生物灭蚊蚴措施。实施措施前要做好充足的准备，除了购买设备、试剂，培训工作人员外，还需要在村里大力宣传以争取民众更多的支持、调查村内村周的各种水体以测算 Bs 用量、调查成蚊和孑孓密度为后期的效果评价提供参考数据。2007 年 8 月至 10 月，每半月使用 Bs 悬浮剂喷洒一次村内和村周各种水体，每平方米水面 Bs 的用量是 8ml。喷洒后中华按蚊幼虫数量下降75.6% ～ 100%，成蚊数量下降 56% ～ 100%，发病率较上年下降 51.3%，事实证明，Bs 生物灭蚊蚴措施有效控制了疟疾传播，减少了疟疾发病。

小提示

1. 生物灭蚊蚴的优势

（1）Bs 生物灭蚊蚴相较于传统化学控制方法来讲，对环境和人类都更为安全，在推荐剂量下对其他昆虫、鱼类、鸟类、哺乳动物和人类无害；

（2）在蚊子对化学杀虫剂产生抗药性的地方，生物灭蚊蚴的防治优势更为突出；

（3）从成本因素考虑，花费不会过于昂贵，与其他蚊媒干预措施相当。

2. 生物灭蚊蚴的可行性

普遍认为有季节性出现或相对较少、界限分明且易于接近的幼虫栖息地的地区，同时人口密度高到足以重复处理繁殖地的地区，控制蚊幼的方法可能最有效，最具成本效益，而这种环境在撒哈拉以南的非洲地区很常见。通过既往的研究报告，非洲常见的传疟按蚊对 Bs 以及苏云金杆菌的以色列亚种（Bti）高度敏

Extended Reading

In the early 20th century, people noticed that mosquitoes were susceptible to certain bacterial pathogens, which sometimes caused endemics in natural populations of larvae. However, as chemical insecticides developed, the biological control method using bacteria against mosquitoes gradually fell out of favor. In the 1960s, Kellen et al. isolated a *Bacillus sphaericus* (Bti) from the fourth instar larvae of *Culiseta incidents*, which can invade healthy larvae through the digestive tract and cause deadly effects on several types of mosquitoes. The biological killing of mosquito larvae has achieved significant results in urban mosquito killing. Since the 1980s, Bti and Bs have been used for mosquito killing in the upper reaches of the Rhine River in Germany for more than 10 consecutive years, with the mosquito population density decreasing by 90% annually, becoming a successful example of biological mosquito killing.

3.4　What are the Tips for Malaria Prevention?

Avoiding bites from *Anopheles* mosquitoes is the most direct and effective measure for preventing malaria. Using insect repellents, bed nets, wearing long-sleeved clothes and long pants while working outdoors, can prevent malaria by reducing the risk of mosquito bites by *Anopheles* mosquitoes. Prophylactic medication is a practical protective measure for populations entering malaria-endemic regions during the *Anopheles* mosquito activity season, with piperaquine phosphate and chloroquine phosphate being common prophylactic medicines. Given the potential risk of malaria infection in endemic regions, it is essential to know whether the destination is a malaria-endemic region before traveling abroad, and to use nets, repellents, and other protective measures when living in highly malaria-endemic regions.

1. Personal application of repellents

Repellents are applied to the body to repel mosquitoes, such as common products like floral water and wind medicated oil. They can be applied to exposed skin such as arms, face, neck, and calves, with a typically effective duration of four hours. Reapplication is necessary after this time. The protection efficacy of these repellents depends on individuals activity level and sweat rate. If one stays

感，那么生物灭蚊蚴能成为非洲地区疟疾控制的有效工具。

3. 生物灭蚊蚴的推广

非洲地区生物灭蚊蚴的实施可以结合中国经验，通过以下几个方面进行推广。

（1）确立对蚊幼虫源管理规划的政策支持；

（2）基线绘制和数据收集，包括幼虫栖息地的水体栖息地和幼虫及成虫的种群数据；

（3）当地工作人员的培训；

（4）多方宣传，提高社区意识。

📖 拓展阅读

20世纪初，人们就注意到蚊子易受到某些细菌病原体的攻击，这些病原体有时可能在自然种群的幼虫中导致流行病，但是随着化学杀虫剂的发展，利用细菌对蚊子进行生物学控制的方法逐渐受到冷落。到20世纪60年代，凯伦等从 *Culiseta incidents* 的四龄幼虫中分离出一种球形芽孢杆菌 (Bs)，能够通过消化道入侵健康幼虫，并对几种蚊子都产生致命性的作用。生物灭蚊蚴措施在城市灭蚊方面取得了显著成效；20世纪80年代开始，在德国的莱茵河上游连续10多年采用Bti和Bs灭蚊蚴，蚊虫种群密度每年下降90%，成为生物灭蚊的成功典范。

3.4 疟疾预防小妙招有哪些？

小提示

避免按蚊叮咬是预防疟疾最简便有效的措施。通过使用驱避剂或蚊帐，野外工作穿长袖衣裤等措施避免被按蚊叮咬可预防疟疾。预防服药是对在按蚊活动季节进入疟疾流行区人群的实用保护性措施，预防药物有磷酸哌喹和磷酸氯喹等。进入疟疾流行区居住就存在感染疟疾可能，因此赴国外前应了解目的地是不是疟疾流行区，赴疟疾高度流行区居住应使用蚊帐、驱蚊剂等防护品。

outdoors, the effective duration of the drug may be shortened, hence timely reapplication is necessary. Tests have shown that the most effective mosquito repellent products currently available mainly contain DEET and insect repellent ingredients, while other products are either completely ineffective or shown with weak effects. The best method for protecting infants and young children from mosquito bites is to use nets. It is also essential to pay attention to allergic reactions to mosquito bites.

Not all mosquitoes are nocturnal creatures; for instance, the *aedes albopictus*, which transmits dengue fever, generally prefers to be active during the day. Therefore, it is essential to prevent mosquito bites during daytime as well. When engaging in outdoor activities in greenbelts, woodlands, and other such regions, it is recommended to use mosquito repellent liquids (repellents) and to dress in light-colored clothes.

2. Remove mosquito breeding sites and killing adult and larval mosquitoes

In addition to commonly known measures like cleaning drains and removing weeds, addressing water accumulation is of importance, as mosquitoes lay eggs and grow freely there. By dealing with water accumulation, not only can the source of mosquitoes, but also the cost of insecticides and labor for killing larvae can be reduced. Unused containers, both indoors and outdoors, as well as in flower beds, should be turned over and placed upside down to prevent water accumulation and mosquito breeding. It is advised to wash the inside of these containers thoroughly before using to remove any eggs that may have been deposited. Common indoor items such as vases and spittoons can also be mosquito breeding sites due to small accumulations of water. Unpredictable places like the water trays under water dispensers can also harbor mosquito larvae, so they should not be overlooked.

3. Long-Lasting Insecticidal Net (LLIN) and Insecticide-Treated Nets (ITN)

Long-lasting insecticidal nets are highly effective mosquito bite prevention products recommended by the WHO for combating malaria in Africa. The material recommended by the WHO is polyethylene or polyester, commonly known as mesh fabric. These materials resemble regular nets but are unique due to their incorporation of such as insecticides pyrethroid, which provide a physical barrier against mosquitoes without harming humans. The insecticides used are resistant to washing. The WHO's current technical standards are that the mosquito knockdown rate reaches 95% and the mosquito mortality rate reaches 80% after a minimum of 20 washes.

1. 个人涂抹驱避剂

驱避剂是为了驱赶蚊子而往身上涂抹的药物，例如常见的有花露水、风油精等，可涂抹于裸露的皮肤处，如手臂、脸颈、小腿等部位，一般4小时内有效，过了这个时间就需要重新涂抹。这些驱避剂的防护效果与个体的活动量、出汗量有关。如果在户外，药效持续时间可能会缩短，应及时补涂。经测试发现，目前最有效的驱蚊产品仍以含有避蚊胺和驱蚊酯成分为主，其他产品不是完全无效就是效果微弱。婴幼儿防蚊最好的方法还是使用蚊帐。另外，要注意观察自己是否有蚊虫叮咬过敏现象。

不是所有蚊子都是夜行动物，比如传播登革热的白纹伊蚊一般就喜欢在白天活动，因此白天外出活动同样需要防蚊。在绿化带、林带或其他类似场所进行户外活动时，最好使用驱蚊液（驱避剂），且尽量穿浅色衣物。

2. 清除蚊虫滋生地与杀灭蚊虫的成虫和幼虫

除了大家所了解的要清理下水道、除杂草等外，最应该引起重视的是处理积水问题，因为蚊虫在那里产卵且自由生长。处理了它不仅可以大大减少蚊虫的来源，也可以节省杀灭幼虫的药物和人力。户内外及花圃中闲置不用的各类容器都应当翻转倒放，以防积水而生蚊。最好在使用前彻底清洁容器内部，以消灭虫卵。室内常见的插花瓶、痰盂等因为有小积水也可能是蚊虫的滋生地。还有一些令人意想不到的地方，比如饮水机的接水盘同样是蚊幼虫的栖身场所，不要掉以轻心。

3. 长效药物蚊帐（LLIN）和药浸蚊帐（ITN）

长效药物蚊帐是由世界卫生组织（WHO）推荐的一种在非洲高效防蚊叮咬的产品。世卫组织推荐的材质为聚乙烯或涤纶，俗称网布。这些布料与普通蚊帐无异。但这种蚊帐的特性是使蚊帐网布含有拟除虫菊酯类等杀虫剂，达到驱杀蚊虫的目的且对人体无害。杀虫剂具有抗洗涤的效果。世卫组织目

Sleeping under insecticide-treated nets can reduce contact between mosquitoes and humans, providing both a physical barrier and insecticidal effects. Increasing the proportion of access to and use of these nets in a community, combined with large-scale mosquito and insect killing, can provide better and more effective protection for the entire community.

4. Indoor residual spraying of insecticides

Indoor residual spraying is another effective measure formulated based on the characteristics of *Anopheles* mosquitoes, which are the vectors of malaria. This involves spraying insecticides inside houses, generally once or twice a year. To strengthen community protection, the coverage of indoor residual spraying should be expanded. Furthermore, individuals can purchase mosquito-repelling and mosquito-killing products that are commercially available in authorized stores, such as mosquito coils, electric mosquito repellent mats (liquids), and insecticidal aerosols.

📖 Extended Reading

Merits and Demerits of DDT

DDT, a widely known organic chlorine pesticide introduced in 1942, was discovered by Swiss chemist Paul Miller, who was awarded the Nobel Prize for his work. The use of DDT has once brought tremendous benefits to humanity. In the early 1930s, its insecticidal properties were discovered, and during World War II, it was used as a secret military supply by the military department to prevent the spread of infectious diseases caused by parasites. DDT played an important role in controlling the endemic of these diseases and improving human health. Later, it was widely used as an insecticide for agricultural pest control, successfully controlling a series of devastating insect pests and contributing to high and stable agricultural yields. However, people soon found that DDT had almost damaged every corner of the earth. It could cause infertility in white rats, kill fish eggs as soon as they hatched, and cause poisoning incidents in livestock and poultry. Within the ecosystem, DDT spread everywhere along the food chain. Plants inevitably absorbed some DDT, and animals also inevitably ingested DDT from the inside and surface of plants, causing harm.

5. Prophylactic medicines

Anti-malaria drugs mainly include piperaquine phosphate and chloroquine phosphate. Chloroquine is the preferred prophylactic drug for adults. In regions with chloroquine-resistant malaria, mefloquine can be used, and pyrimethamine or doxycycline also. Pregnant women and children should consider chloroquine

前的技术指标为 20 次洗涤后，蚊虫击倒率为 95%，蚊虫死亡率为 80%。

睡在有药浸蚊帐保护的床上可以减少蚊虫与人体之间的接触，因为它提供了物理屏障，且具有杀虫效果。在一个社区内，提高获取和使用这种蚊帐的比率，加上大规模杀灭蚊虫，可以对整个社区的人口予以更好、更有效的保护。

4. 室内滞留喷洒杀虫剂

室内滞留喷洒是根据疟疾传播媒介按蚊的特性而制定的又一有效措施。这涉及使用杀虫剂喷洒房屋的内部，一般一年一次或两次。当然，为了加大对社区的保护力度，应使室内滞留喷洒的覆盖面达到相当程度。此外，家庭室内使用防蚊灭蚊的方法还可到正规商场购买上市的产品，如蚊香或电热灭蚊片（液）、杀虫气雾剂等。

📖 **拓展阅读**

DDT 的功与过

人们很熟悉的 DDT，是 1942 年面世的一种有机氯农药。瑞士化学家保罗·米勒因发明 DDT 而获诺贝尔奖。DDT 的使用曾给人类带来巨大的福利。20 世纪 30 年代初期，人们便发现 DDT 的杀虫效用。在第二次世界大战期间，它作为保密的军事物资被军事部门用来防制传染疾病的害虫。对于控制这些传染病的流行，增进人类的健康，它起了重要的作用，后来 DDT 用来作为防制农作物害虫的一种杀虫剂被广泛地使用，它成功使一系列毁灭性虫害得到了控制，对农业的高产稳产作出了贡献。但人们很快发现，DDT 几乎侵害了地球上每一个角落的生命。它能引起大白鼠不孕，使鱼的受精卵一孵化就死去，它造成家畜、家禽的中毒事故。在生物世界内部，DDT 沿着食物链扩散到四面八方。植物不可避免地吸收一部分 DDT。动物也难免把植物体内和表面的 DDT 吃入肚内，引起危害。

---

5. 预防药物

抗疟药物主要包括磷酸哌喹和磷酸氯喹等。成人预防性药物首选氯喹，在耐氯喹疟疾流行区，可选用甲氟喹，也可选用乙胺嘧啶或多西环素。孕妇

as the first-line drug for malaria prevention. Pyrimethamine has an inhibitory effect falciparum malaria and vivax malaria and is the preferred drug for etiologic prophylaxis. It can also prevent the sporozoite proliferation of malaria parasites in mosquitoes, thus controlling the spread of the disease. Combining drug interventions with vaccination will greatly reduce the incidence and mortality of malaria. However, the diversity of malaria parasite antigens poses significant challenges for vaccine development. Drug prophylaxis is currently a commonly used measure.

For travelers, chemical prophylaxis can suppress malaria, achieving the purpose of disease prevention. For pregnant women living in moderately to highly endemic regions, the WHO recommends using sulfadoxine-pyrimethamine for at least three doses of intermittent preventive therapy after the first three months of pregnancy. Similarly, for infants living in highly endemic regions of Africa, it is recommended to receive three doses of sulfadoxine-pyrimethamine intermittent preventive therapy simultaneously with routine vaccination.

3.5　How can the Malaria Endemics be Recognized?

Let's rewind to the early 21st century, on a hot June afternoon, in a northern county of central China. The scorching sun beat down on the fields, where people were busy harvesting wheat. A middle-aged woman rode to the village health clinic in a battery-powered three-wheeled vehicle, dragging a man covered with a blanket, urgently asking the elderly village doctor to diagnose her husband's strange illness. The doctor and the woman worked together to lift the patient into the clinic and asked about his condition. The woman replied, "My husband has started shivering again, just like he did two days ago. First, he was so cold that even covering himself with winter quilts couldn't help. Then he became feverish, sweat profusely, and after the sweat passed, he felt exhausted and fell asleep. Yesterday, he was fine all day, and I thought he was recovering from a cold. But why is he worse today after lunch? He can't even get up!" The doctor quickly took the patient's temperature, which read 40° C! The elderly doctor said, "He is 'Da Bai Zi'" (footnote: malaria is locally known as "Da Bai Zi"). This season, this disease is common in our area. Testing blood at the township health center can help confirm if it's malaria. The center has specific medicine that can cure it once taken. Don't worry too much. The woman hurried to the township health center, which was two

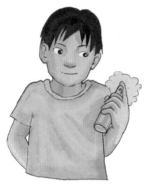

个人涂抹驱避剂
Personal application of repellents

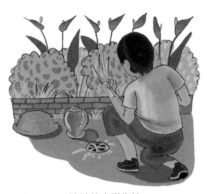

清除蚊虫滋生地
Remove mosquito breeding sites

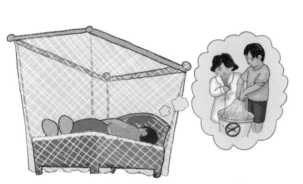

使用药浸蚊帐
Using insecticide-treated nets

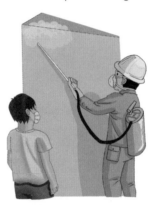

室内滞留喷洒杀虫剂
Indoor residual spraying of insecticides

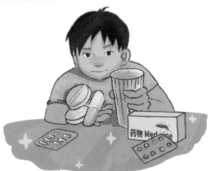

提前服用预防药物
Taking prophylactic drugs in advance

图 3-4　疟疾预防小妙招
Figure 3-4　Tips for Malaria Prevention

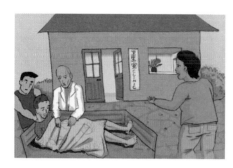
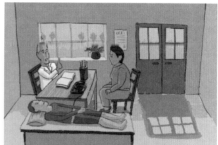
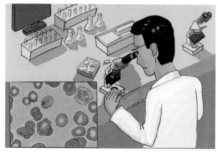
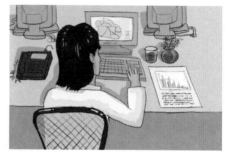
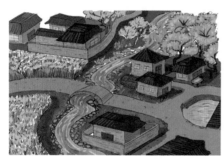
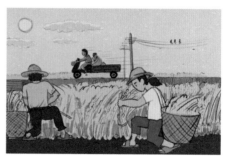

图 3-5　小村镇发现了疟疾病例
Figure 3-5　Malaria cases were found in small villages and towns

miles away.

The elderly doctor called the disease prevention and control department of the township health center: "We have had three suspected malaria patients in our village in the past week, including the one just transferred to your center. This disease hasn't been seen in a long time, but now it's becoming more common. Shouldn't you send someone from the endemic prevention station to check out what's going on in our village?"

At the township health center's laboratory, a doctor was examining the blood smear of the male patient transferred from the village. Under the microscope, the

儿童宜服用氯喹作为预防首选。乙胺嘧啶对恶性疟和间日疟有抑制作用，是病因性预防的首选药；其还能阻止疟原虫在蚊体内的孢子增殖，起控制传播的作用。疟疾的药物干预与预防接种相结合，将有望大大降低疟疾的发病率和死亡率。但疟原虫抗原的多样性给疫苗研制带来很大的困难。药物预防是目前较常用的措施。

就旅行者而言，可以通过化学预防来抑制疟疾，达到防病目的。对于生活在中度至高度传播地区的孕妇，世卫组织建议在妊娠前 3 个月之后的每次预定产前检查时，使用磺胺多辛-乙胺嘧啶进行至少 3 剂间歇性预防治疗。同样，对于生活在非洲高传播地区的婴儿，建议在常规疫苗接种的同时，进行 3 剂磺胺多辛-乙胺嘧啶间歇性预防治疗。

3.5 怎么知道发生了疟疾流行？

时间回到 21 世纪初一个酷热的 6 月的下午，在中国一个中部省北部县，骄阳似火，收麦子的人们在地里忙碌着。一名中年妇女骑着电动三轮车，拉着一个盖着被子的男人来到了村卫生室，一脸焦急地让老村医看看她丈夫得了什么怪病，老村医与其合力将患者抬进屋询问病情，妇女答："我丈夫又开始发冷了，前天下午也是这样，先冷得要命，把冬天的被子盖着都受不了，然后发热，出了好多汗，出过汗就累得睡着了，昨天一天没事，以为是感冒好了，咋今天吃过中饭后又开始啦，还更重了，人都起不来了？！"赶紧量下体温，40℃！老村医说道："他这是'打摆子'，这个季节我们这儿就好得这个病，去镇卫生院验个血就能确定是不是了，镇卫生院有特效药，一吃就好了，不要太担心。"女人赶紧带着男人去了二里地外的镇卫生院。

老村医给镇卫生院防保科打电话："我们村这一个星期接连有 3 个疑似疟疾患者了，刚才过去你们那儿一个，这个病有好多年没怎么看到了，咋又多

malaria parasites, which haven't been seen in years, appear in dense clusters. A slide box nearby contained positive blood smears from this month. The number collected that month has already exceeded the total for all of last year.

The doctor in charge of reporting endemics at the township health center counts the number of malaria cases — seven in just one week in this township, spread across three villages. Meanwhile, a doctor from the county disease prevention and control center has analyzed the case numbers for this year and last year. The data shows that the number of malaria cases in the county has significantly increased compared to last week and the same period last year, indicating a localized malaria outbreak.

3.6 What are the Characteristics of Malaria Epidemic?

Tips

Malaria is predominantly endemic in several regions worldwide, including Africa, Southeast Asia, the Eastern Mediterranean, and the Americas, among which sub-Saharan Africa and Southeast Asia exhibit a high prevalence of malaria. Currently, China has thousands of imported malaria cases annually from these endemic regions, such as Africa and Southeast Asia, and the transmission vectors still exist in China. Therefore, China is still at risk of malaria re-establishment after importation.

📖 Extended Reading

The malaria situation is particularly severe in the Sub-Saharan Africa, with most cases and deaths occurring in those countries. However, the WHO regions of Southeast Asia, Eastern Mediterranean, Western Pacific, and Americas also face great dangers. In 2022, of the 85 countries where malaria is endemic, 29 countries accounted for 95% of global malaria cases. Nigeria (27%), the Democratic Republic of the Congo (12%), Uganda (5%), Mozambique (4%) and Niger (3%) accounted for approximately 51% of all global cases. Nigeria (23%), the Democratic Republic of the Congo (11%), the United Republic of Tanzania (5%), Burkina Faso (4%), Mozambique (4%) and Niger (4%) accounted for approximately 51% of all global cases in 2022. Malaria prevalence differs between regions, with falciparum malaria dominant in Africa, Papua New Guinea, and South Pacific island countries, and vivax malaria dominant in America, Middle East, and most parts of Asia.

起来了？！你们要不要让防疫站的同志来我们这儿看看咋回事了？"

镇卫生院化验室，一名医生正在查验刚才从村里转诊来的男性患者的血涂片，显微镜下多年未见的疟原虫这一段期间密集来报到，显微镜旁摆着一个玻片盒，里面收集了这个月的阳性血涂片，这一个月收集的已经超过去年一年的总数了。

镇卫生院负责上报疫情的医生正统计着疟疾病例数，这个镇一个星期就报告了 7 个病例，分布在 3 个村。同时，县疾病预防控制中心的医生已经将今年与去年的病例数进行了统计分析，显示：本周全县疟疾病例数明显高于上周及去年同期水平，疟疾呈局部流行态势。

3.6 疟疾流行特征有哪些?

小提示

疟疾流行区主要分布在非洲、东南亚、东地中海和美洲地区，其中撒哈拉以南的非洲和东南亚地区疟疾高度流行。目前我国每年有上千例从非洲、东南亚等疟疾流行地区回国的输入性病例，而我国传疟媒介依然存在，因此我国仍面临着境外疟疾输入后再传播的风险。

拓展阅读

撒哈拉沙漠以南的非洲疫情较严重，且大多数疟疾病例和死亡都发生在那些国家。然而，世卫组织的东南亚、东地中海、西太平洋和美洲区域也危机四伏。在 2022 年疟疾流行的 85 个国家中，29 个国家的病例数占全球疟疾病例总数的 95%。尼日利亚（27%）、刚果民主共和国（12%）、乌干达（5%）、莫桑比克（4%）和尼日尔（3%）约占全球所有病例的 51%。尼日利亚（23%）、刚果民主共和国（11%）、坦桑尼亚联合共和国（5%）、布基纳法索（4%）、莫桑比克（4%）和尼日尔（4%）约占 2022 年全球疟疾死亡总数的 51%。疟疾流行在不同地区有所不同，非洲以及巴布亚新几内亚和南太平洋岛

In 2022, the WHO African region accounted for about 93.6% of global malaria cases and 95.4% of deaths, with 78.1% of deaths occurring in children under 5 years old. From 2019 to 2020, the estimated malaria cases in this region rose from 218 million to 230 million, and deaths from 552,000 to 604,000. From 2020 to 2022, the estimated malaria cases in the region remained almost unchanged, while the number of deaths was reduced to 580,000. However, from 2019 to 2022, the estimated number of malaria cases increased substantially.

In 2022, 9 malaria endemic countries in the WHO Southeast Asian region reported 5.2 million cases, accounting for 2% of the global malaria burden. In 2022, India alone accounted for approximately 65.7% of all malaria cases in the region, and more than one-third of cases were caused by *Plasmodium vivax*. Malaria cases have decreased by 78% over the past 20 years, from 22.8 million cases in 2000 to 5.2 million in 2020, and the incidence decreased by 83%, from 17.6 cases per 1,000 people to 3 cases. Sri Lanka was certified as malaria-free in 2016.

The WHO Eastern Mediterranean region witnessed a 38% reduction in malaria cases from 2000 to 2015, but experienced a steady 92% increase from 2016 to 2020! In just 2021 to 2022,Pakistan, Afghanistan, and Sudan reported estimated increases of 2,100,000, 94,000, and 35,000 malaria cases, respectively. In 2022, approximately 29.4% of cases were caused by *Plasmodium vivax*, chiefly in Afghanistan and Pakistan. The region's estimated increase in malaria deaths was primarily in Sudan, where more than 80% of cases were caused by *Plasmodium falciparum*. Although malaria deaths decreased by about 45% in the region, Afghanistan, Pakistan, and Yemen experienced slight reductions. However, virtually all deaths were attributed to malaria.

The number of malaria cases in the Western Pacific region of the WHO decreased from 2.6 million in 2000 to 1.9 million in 2022, a reduction of 48%. The number of malaria-related deaths also fell significantly by 56%. The increase in cases and deaths from 2021 to 2022 was primarily due to the increase in case numbers in Papua New Guinea. Over time, the proportion of cases caused by *Plasmodium vivax* in the region has increased to some extent. From 2020 to 2022, there was a significant increase in malaria cases in Solomon Islands and Ghana. The proportion of cases of *Plasmodium* vivax in the region increased from 17% in 2000 to 27% in 2022. Papua New Guinea accounted for 90% of all malaria cases in the region, followed by Solomon Islands, Cambodia, Tanzania, and the Philippines. Since 2017, there have been no domestic malaria cases in China, and it was certified malaria-free in 2021. Malaysia also has not reported any human malaria cases for 5 consecutive years, but it reported 2500 cases caused by *Plasmodium knowlesi* in 2022.

国主要流行恶性疟;而美洲、中东、亚洲大部分国家和地区主要流行间日疟。

2022 年,世卫组织非洲区域约占全球病例数的 93.6% 和死亡人数的 95.4%;该区域 78.1% 的死亡是 5 岁以下儿童。2019 年至 2020 年,该区域估计疟疾病例从 2.18 亿增加到 2.3 亿,死亡人数从 55.2 万人增加到 60.4 万人。2020 年至 2022 年期间,该区域的估计病例数几乎没有变化,而死亡人数减少到 58 万。然而,在 2019 至 2022 年期间,估计病例数大幅增加。

2022 年,世卫组织东南亚区域有 9 个疟疾流行国家,出现 520 万病例,占全球疟疾病例负担的 2%。2022 年,印度约占该区域所有疟疾病例的 65.7%;该地区超过三分之一的病例是由间日疟原虫引起的。在过去 20 年中,疟疾病例减少了 78%,从 2000 年的 2 280 万例减少到 2022 年的 520 万例,发病率也减少了 83%,从每千人 17.6 例减少到每千人 3 例。斯里兰卡于 2016 年被认证为无疟疾国家。

世卫组织东地中海区域的疟疾病例在 2000 年至 2015 年期间减少了 38%,但在 2016 年至 2022 年期间反而稳步增加了 92%!仅 2021 年至 2022 年,巴基斯坦、阿富汗和苏丹 3 个国家估计疟疾病例分别增加 210 万例、94 000 例和 35 000 例。2022 年约 29.4% 的病例是由间日疟原虫引起的,主要发生在阿富汗和巴基斯坦。该区域估计疟疾死亡人数的增加主要在苏丹,那里 80% 以上的病例是由恶性疟原虫造成的。虽然疟疾死亡人数在该区域减少了约 45%,阿富汗、巴基斯坦、也门也稍有减少。但几乎所有死亡病例都是因为疟疾。

世卫组织西太平洋区域的疟疾病例从 2000 年的 260 万例减少到 2022 年的 190 万例,减少了 48%。疟疾死亡人数也显著下降了 56%。2021 年至 2022 年期间病例和死亡人数的增加主要是由于巴布亚新几内亚国家病例数的增加。随着时间的推移,该区域由间日疟原虫造成的病例比例有所增加。2020 年至 2022 年期间,所罗门群岛和加纳的病例显著增加。随着时间的推移,该区域间日疟病例的比例有所增加,从 2000 年的 17% 左右增加到 2022 年的

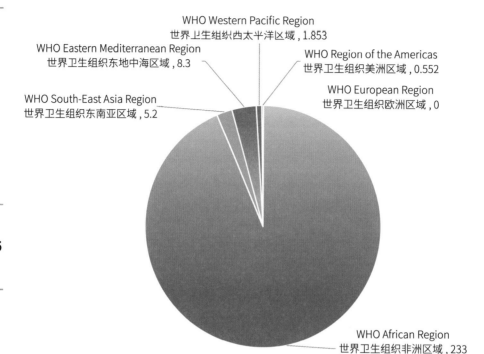

数据来源：世界卫生组织 2023 年世界疟疾报告
Source: World malaria report 2023

图 3-6　2022 年世界卫生组织各区域估计疟疾病例数（百万）
Figure 3-6　Estimated malaria cases in the WHO Regions in 2022 (million)

From 2000 to 2022, the number of malaria cases and case incidences decreased by 64% and 72% respectively in the WHO American region. Paraguay, Argentina, El Salvador and Belize were certified malaria-free in 2018, 2019, 2021 and 2023, respectively. The region has few malaria-related deaths, with an estimated number of 343 deaths in 2022, most of whom were adults.

Countries with no domestic cases for at least 3 consecutive years are considered to have eliminated malaria. In 2022, Iran and Malaysia reported no indigenous cases for 5 consecutive years, as did Belize and Cape Verde for the third year. After 4 years with no malaria cases, China and El Salvador were certified malaria-free in 2021. As of the end of 2023, a total of 15 countries worldwide had been certified as malaria-free by the WHO.

27%。巴布亚新几内亚占该区域所有病例的 90%，其次是所罗门群岛、柬埔寨、坦桑尼亚和菲律宾。自 2017 年以来，中国没有出现本土疟疾病例，并于 2021 年被认定为无疟疾国家。马来西亚也已连续 5 年没有出现人类疟疾病例，但在 2022 年报告了 2 500 例由诺氏疟原虫引发的病例。

2000 年至 2022 年期间，在世卫组织美洲区域，疟疾病例和病例发生率分别下降了 64% 和 72%。巴拉圭、阿根廷、萨尔瓦多和伯利兹分别于 2018 年、2019 年、2021 年和 2023 年被认证为无疟疾国家。该区域与疟疾相关的死亡人数很少，2022 年估计有 343 人死亡，其中大多数是成年人。

本地病例至少连续 3 年为零的国家被认为已经消除了疟疾。2022 年，伊朗和马来西亚连续 5 年报告本土病例为零，伯利兹和佛得角第 3 年报告本土病例为零。继 4 年零疟疾病例之后，中国和萨尔瓦多于 2021 年被认证为无疟疾国家。截至 2023 年年底，全世界共有 15 个国家被世卫组织认证为无疟疾国家。

3.7 案例 5 中国卫生奇迹——爱国卫生运动

爱国卫生运动是人类卫生发展史上的一项伟大创举和成功实践，被世界卫生组织称为"中国的卫生奇迹"，是中国公共卫生工作的重要组成部分，在中国已经有近 70 年历史，是中国持续时间最长的群众性运动。其主要目的为调动广大人民群众，全民动员、全民参与，不断改善城乡环境，着力解决突出的卫生问题，普及健康生活方式。世界卫生组织指出，远在"健康融入所有政策"成为全球口号之前，中国就已通过爱国卫生运动践行着这一原则；远在"健康城市"理念诞生之前，爱国卫生运动就已通过更好的环境和个人卫生创造了它们。2013 年和 2017 年，世界卫生组织先后授予中国政府"健康（卫生）城市特别奖"和"社会健康治理杰出典范奖"，表彰中国爱国卫生运动取得的成就。

3.7 Case 5 The Health Miracle of China — Patriotic Public Health Campaign

The Patriotic Public Health Campaign is a pioneering and successful in the history of human health development, which has been called "The Health Miracle of the People's Republic of China" by the WHO. It is an important part of China's public health work and has a history of nearly 70 years in China. It is the longest-lasting mass campaign in China, aiming at mobilizing and involving the entire population in improving urban and rural environments, focusing on addressing prominent health issues, and promoting healthy lifestyles. The WHO states that China had already implemented the principle of "Health in All Policies" through the Patriotic Public Health Campaign, long before it became a global slogan. Furthermore, long before the concept of "Healthy City" was born, the Patriotic Public Health Campaign had created them through better environmental and personal hygiene. In 2013 and 2017, the WHO granted the Chinese government the "Special Award for Healthy (Health) City" and the "Outstanding Model Award for Social Health Governance" respectively, recognizing the achievements of the Patriotic Public Health Campaign in China.

From 1949 to 1952, a nationwide mass health campaign was initiated to address unsanitary conditions and the widespread prevalence of infectious diseases. Within just half a year, the country removed over 15 million tons of waste, cleaned up 280,000 kilometers of channels, built or renovated 4.9 million toilets, and renovated 1.3 million water wells. A total of over 44 million mice were caught, and over 2 million kilograms of mosquitoes, flies, and fleas were eradicated. Moreover, numerous dirty puddles were filled in, and the sanitary conditions of vast urban and rural regions improved to varying degrees. In the winter of 1955, the state proposed combining the Patriotic Public Health Campaign with the "Eradicating the Four Pests" ① and promoting hygiene. The Patriotic Public Health Campaign played a positive and effective role in preventing and controlling zoonotic diseases, malaria and other mosquito-borne infectious and endemic diseases, and guaranteeing public health. It has enabled China to withstand severe tests of various endemics such as plague, smallpox, cholera, schistosomiasis, and malaria under the circumstances of "poverty and blankness" .

---

① page note: four pests refer to rats, sparrows, flies, and mosquitoes, and later sparrows were replaced by cockroaches.

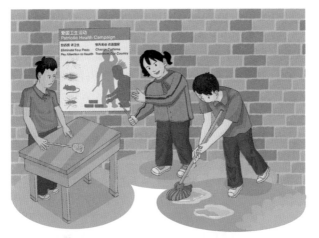

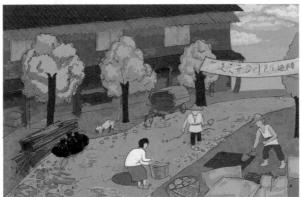

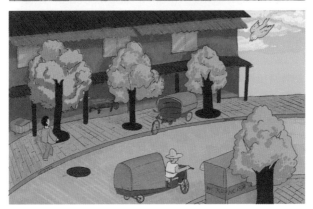

图 3-7　开展爱国卫生运动，清洁家园除四害
Figure 3-7　Carrying out Patriotic Health Campaign, Cleaning Home and Eradicating Four Pests

Carrying out the Patriotic Public Health Campaign is not merely a simple cleaning effort. The evolution of times has expanded the scope of the Patriotic Public Health Campaign, encompassing the improvement of human settlements, dietary habits, social mental health, and public health facilities, which are integral components. In 1982, "launching mass health activities" was written into the Constitution, establishing the legal status of the Patriotic Public Health Campaign. Locally, the "Two Management and Five Improvements" work was advanced, focusing on "managing water and feces, improving water wells, toilets, animal pens, stoves, and the environment." In 1989, the National Health Town Creation Campaign was initiated, producing a number of national health cities and towns and significantly improving the urban and rural environmental appearance. At the beginning of the 21st century, in response to sudden and significant epidemics such as SARS and avian influenza, the "Three Focuses and One Fostering" Campaign was launched in various places, focusing on civilization, hygiene, science, and fostering new customs. The "Three Clearances and Three Improvements" environmental cleanup, which involves clearing sludge, garbage, and roadblocks, as well as improving water facilities, toilets, and roads, has been vigorously pursued. These initiatives have made positive contributions to ensuring the health of the general public. In 2017, the guiding principles of the Patriotic Public Health Campaign in the new era were proposed, namely "people's health-centric, government-led, inter-departmental collaboration, whole-society mobilization, prevention-oriented, mass prevention and control, scientific management by law, and joint construction and sharing by the whole people." Through the creation of national health cities and towns, the average incidence of notifiable infectious diseases was reduced by 19.4%, the proportion of standardized markets increased from 35.2% to 60.6%, and the residents' satisfaction rate with the urban appearance environment increased from 30% to 98%. The satisfaction rate of the effect of establishing healthy cities and towns was up to 98%, which achieved good economic and social benefits. By the end of 1995, the number of people benefiting from the national water improvement project reached 779 million, accounting for 97.03% of the rural population. Among them, 43.51% of the rural population gained access to tap water, effectively eradicating diseases such as Keshan disease and Kaschin-Beck disease. These efforts have contributed to the prevention of diseases, safeguarded health, developed rural economy, and improved the quality of life for farmers. Over the years, the Patriotic Public Health Campaign has carried out mass health campaigns such as "Clean Your Homeland and Prevent Mosquito-Borne Diseases,"

1949 年至 1952 年，为了改变不卫生状况和传染病严重流行的现实，在全国普遍开展了群众性卫生运动。仅半年里，全国就清除垃圾 1 500 多万吨，疏通渠道 28 万公里，新建改建厕所 490 万个，改建水井 130 万眼。共捕鼠 4 400 多万只，消灭蚊、蝇、蚤共 200 多万斤。还填平了一大批污水坑塘，广大城乡的卫生面貌有了不同程度的改善。1955 年冬，国家提出把爱国卫生运动和"除四害"①、讲卫生结合起来。爱国卫生运动对防治人畜共患病、防治疟疾等蚊虫传播的传染病和流行病、保障健康起到了积极有效的作用，使中国在"一穷二白"的情况下经受住了鼠疫、天花、霍乱、血吸虫病、疟疾等各类疫情的严峻考验。

开展爱国卫生运动，绝不是简单的清扫工作。时代的变迁赋予了爱国卫生运动不同的内容，改善人居环境、饮食习惯、社会心理健康、公共卫生设施等多个方面都成为其题中应有之意。1982 年，"开展群众性的卫生活动"被写入宪法，确立了爱国卫生运动的法律地位。各地深入推进"管水、粪，改水井、厕所、畜圈、炉灶、环境"的"两管五改"工作。1989 年，启动全国卫生城镇创建活动，打造了一批国家卫生城镇，城乡环境面貌显著改善。21 世纪初，针对非典、禽流感等突发重大疫情，各地开展了"三讲一树"活动——讲文明、讲卫生、讲科学、树新风，推进"三清三改"的环境整治——清污泥、清垃圾、清路障和改水、改厕、改路，为保障人民群众健康作出积极贡献。2017 年提出新时代爱国卫生运动的方针，即"以人民健康为中心，政府主导，跨部门协作，全社会动员，预防为主，群防群控，依法科学治理，全民共建共享"。通过国家卫生城镇创建，法定传染病报告发病率平均降低 19.4%，规范集贸市场比例由 35.2% 提高到 60.6%，居民对市容环境的满意率由 30% 提高到 98%，对创建卫生城镇效果的满意度达到 98%，取得了良好的经济和社

① 四害指老鼠、麻雀、苍蝇、蚊子，后将麻雀改为蟑螂。

strengthened the work of disease vector prevention and control, and achieved the elimination of filariasis and malaria, reducing incidence of schistosomiasis to the lowest level in the history, significantly decreasing the endemic of dengue fever, and successfully combating emerging infectious diseases such as H7N9 influenza and SARS. These efforts have laid an important foundation for the prevention and control of epidemics.

Tips

1. Advantages of Patriotic Health Campaign

(1) Universal participation: significantly enhance the public's self-protection capabilities. It comprehensively advances urban and rural environmental sanitation improvement and addresses shortcomings in public health environments by focusing on key areas and vulnerable points.

(2) Keeping up with the times: promote civilized and healthy lifestyles. Encourage self-discipline and healthy living, practice green and environmental protection concepts, and promote the mental health of the masses.

(3) Internalization: generally improve the health and civilization literacy of the masses.

2. Feasibility of Patriotic Health Campaign

The campaign effectively leverages the coordinating roles of the state, collective entities, and individuals and organize social forces to conduct pest and disease control, eradicate unhealthy habits, enhance social health awareness, transform nature, improve the environment, and eradicate factors that harm health, thus upgrading the quality of life, health literacy, and health levels for the entire nation. This is an effective means for the pest and disease control, disaster prevention, and endemic control, and one of the best ways to enhance social, economic, environmental, and health benefits.

3. Promotion of Patriotic Health Campaign

In essence, the Patriotic Public Health Campaign is a declaration of war against backward lifestyles and habits, carrying the significance of changing customs. The campaign can be promoted and applied in the following five aspects.

(1) Formulating mass health and wellness conventions.

(2) Strengthening general health education.

(3) Launching health reminder columns in the media.

(4) Strengthening health information management by leveraging big data.

(5) Integrating health and wellness behaviors into the legal process.

会效益。至 1995 年年底全国改水受益人口达 7.99 亿，占农村人口的 97.03%；其中 43.51% 的农村人口喝上了自来水，基本消除了克山病、大骨节病。这对预防疾病，保障健康，发展农村经济，改善农民生活质量都发挥了积极作用。多年来，爱国卫生运动开展"清洁家园、灭蚊防病"等群众卫生运动，加强病媒生物防制工作，消除了丝虫病和疟疾，血吸虫病疫情降至历史最低水平，登革热疫情明显下降，成功抗击了 H7N9 流感、SARS 等突发传染病疫情，为疫情防控打下了重要基础。

小提示

1. 爱国卫生运动的优势

（1）全民参与，大幅提升群众自我防护能力。以重点场所、薄弱环节为重点，全面推进城乡环境卫生综合整治，补齐公共卫生环境短板。

（2）与时俱进，提倡文明健康的生活方式。倡导自主自律的健康生活，践行绿色环保的生活理念，促进群众心理健康。

（3）内化于心，群众健康文明素养普遍提升。

2. 爱国卫生运动的可行性

发挥国家、集体、个人的协调作用，组织社会力量，除害灭病、革除陋习，增强社会卫生意识，改造自然、改善环境、消除危害健康的因素，提高全民生活质量、卫生素质及健康水平。爱国卫生运动是除害灭病、抗灾防疫的有效手段，是提高社会效益、经济效益、环境效益、健康效益的极佳途径之一。

3. 爱国卫生运动的推广

爱国卫生运动从本质上讲，就是向落后的生活方式和习惯宣战，具有移风易俗的意义。可以从以下五个方面推广应用。

（1）制定群众卫生健康公约。

（2）加强健康通识教育。

（3）媒体推出健康提醒栏目。

（4）依托大数据加强健康信息管理。

（5）将卫生健康行为纳入法治进程。

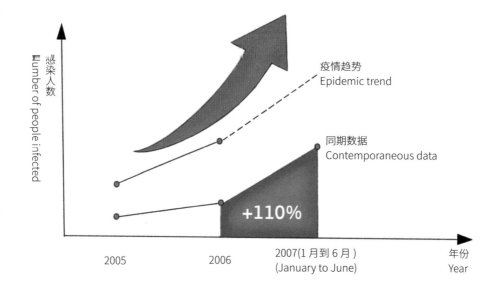

感染人数
Number of people infected

疫情趋势
Epidemic trend

同期数据
Contemporaneous data

+110%

2005   2006   2007(1 月到 6 月)   年份
                              (January to June)   Year

图 3-8　某省疟疾疫情近 3 年内上升
Figure 3-8   Increase in the number of Malaria Cases in Recent 3 Years in X Province

3.8   How Extensive is the Range of Malaria Endemic? Where does it Occur Most Severely?

To understand the prevalence and severity of malaria across the X Province from January to June of 2007, staff from the Provincial Center for Disease Prevention and Control logged into the national surveillance system for disease prevention and infectious diseases, They prepared preparing to collect malaria endemic data and discussed the next steps for malaria prevention and control measures by analyzing the patterns of malaria incidence. In the system, the number of malaria cases and individual case cards of malaria in the counties and districts under the jurisdiction of the province were obtained according to the following query conditions: disease name as malaria (including vivax malaria and unspecified malaria), case type as all (including suspected, clinically diagnosed, and confirmed cases), current address, and onset date between January and June 2007 and the previous two years. The individual case cards included information such as patient name, gender, age, a detailed current address (specific to province, city, county, township, administrative village, and natural village), onset date, diagnosis date, and reporting unit and other information. Statistical analysis of the individual case

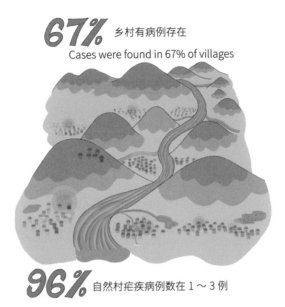

67% 乡村有病例存在
Cases were found in 67% of villages

96% 自然村疟疾病例数在 1 ～ 3 例

In 96% of natural villages,the number of malaria cases was about 1 to 3 cases

图 3-9　疟疾在自然村发生了局部暴发
Figure 3-9　Local Outbreak of Malaria in Natural Villages

3.8　疟疾流行范围有多大？哪里流行最严重？

为了解全省 2007 年 1 月至 6 月疟疾流行范围和流行程度，省疾病预防控制中心工作人员登录国家疾病预防传染病监测系统，准备收集疟疾疫情数据，通过分析疟疾发病特征探讨下一步要采取的疟疾防控措施。在系统中按照以下查询条件：疾病名称为疟疾（包括间日疟和未确诊的疟疾）、病例类型为全部（包括疑似、临床诊断和确诊病例）、现住址、发病日期为 2007 年 1 ～ 6 月及前两年，查询获得该省所辖县区疟疾病例数和疟疾病例个案卡。个案卡中包括病例姓名、性别、年龄、现住详细地址（具体到省市县乡行政村自然村）、发病日期、诊断日期、报告单位等个案信息。通过对病例个案卡统计分析发现，该省近三年疟疾疫情呈上升态势，2007 年 1 ～ 6 月间日疟病例数较

cards revealed that the malaria endemic in the province had been on the rise in recent years. The number of vivax malaria cases in the first half of 2007 increased by 110% compared to the same period of the previous year, and 90% of malaria cases were concentrated in 24 counties and districts, located in the northern region of the province, which is a vivax malaria-endemic region dominated by *Anopheles sinensis* as the sole transmission vector. There are some cases in 67% of villages among these 24 counties and districts, with 1 to 3 cases occurred in 96% of the natural villages. The results showed that there had been a recurrence of vivax malaria and local outbreaks at the village level in some regions of the province, with a wide and scattered distribution of cases. The conclusion drawn was that an outbreak of vivax malaria had occurred in the region, province timely emergency response and intervention measures to curb the outbreak.

3.9 Case 6 Chinese Barefoot Doctor Model—Grass-roots Health Care Security

The barefoot doctors were a unique phenomenon in the history of Chinese health care, having been selected in the 1960s and 1970s to address the lack of medical resources and personnel in rural regions. These rural primary care medical practitioners received only basic medical and nursing training, providing medical insurance for rural residents, but they were not formally employed by the state and lacked official medical qualifications. They were directly supervised and guided by local township health centers, treating common ailments, assisting with childbirth, and focusing on reducing infant mortality and controlling the spread of infectious diseases. Their ranks were primarily drawn from three sources: medical families, short-term trained nursing students, and self-taught individuals with a certain level of nursing ability. By the end of 1977, the number of barefoot doctors had reached over 1.5 million. After 1985, they were transformed into rural doctors, and the term "barefoot doctor" gradually fell out of use. Starting in 2004, rural doctors were licensed to practice after completing relevant registration and training exams, officially ending the era of barefoot doctors. Despite their low salaries, barefoot doctors enjoyed the trust and respect of local rural residents, gaining a good reputation through publicity, with some even becoming household names nationwide. These healthcare practitioners were both farmers and doctors, working in the fields during peak farming seasons and providing medical services during off-

去年同期增加 110%，90% 的疟疾病例集中分布在 24 个县区，这些县区位于该省北部区域，是以中华按蚊为单一传播媒介的间日疟流行区。这 24 个县区中 67% 的乡村有病例存在，其中 96% 的自然村疟疾病例数为 1～3 例。结果显示在该省内部分地区出现间日疟疫情回升和以村为单位的局部高发，病例分布具有广而分散的特点。结论为该区域间日疟高发，须及时采取应急处置措施，遏制疫情暴发。

3.9 案例 6 中国赤脚医生模式——基层医疗卫生保障

赤脚医生是中国卫生史上的一个特殊产物，是 20 世纪 60、70 年代为缓解我国广大农村地区缺医少药的问题而选拔的农村基层兼职医疗人员。赤脚医生只接受了最基本的医疗和护理训练，为农村居民提供医疗保障，没有纳入国家编制，也不是正式医生。赤脚医生受当地乡镇卫生院直接领导和医护指导，可以治疗常见病，能为产妇接生，主要任务是降低婴儿死亡率和控制传染病流行。当时赤脚医生的来源主要有三部分：一是医学世家；二是经医护专业短期培训的学员；三是公认有一定医护能力的自学成才者。到 1977 年年底，赤脚医生数量一度达到 150 多万名。1985 年以后他们转变为乡村医生，赤脚医生的称呼逐渐消失。2004 年以后乡村医生经过相应的注册及培训考试后，以正式医生的名义执照开业，赤脚医生的历史自此结束。虽然赤脚医生的收入不高，但他们得到了当地农村居民的信任和尊重，也通过宣传赢得了好名声，一些模范赤脚医生在全国家喻户晓。他们亦农亦医，农忙时务农，农闲时行医，或是白天务农，晚上行医送药。他们没有固定薪金，许多人要赤着脚，荷锄扶犁耕地种田，农村社员将"半农半医"卫生员亲切称呼为"赤脚医生"。赤脚医生在广大农村地区为普及爱国卫生知识、除"四害"、控制疟疾等传染病流行，做出了巨大贡献。

peak times, or tending to their agricultural duties during the day and distributing medicine and treatments at night. They didn't have a fixed salary, and many of them had to work barefoot, hoeing and plowing farmland. Rural cooperative members referred to these "semi-agricultural and semi-medical" health workers as "barefoot doctors." They made significant contributions to promoting patriotic health knowledge, eradicating four pests, and controlling the spread of malaria and other infectious diseases in rural regions.

During the implementation of the malaria prevention and control program, particularly during severe endemic periods, the implementation of malaria control program relies heavily on the pivotal role played by barefoot doctors. These healthcare workers, deeply rooted in their local communities, organize and execute critical activities such as medication distribution and mosquito killing activities. They either carried medication and water, going door-to-door and deep into the fields, serving each person taking the medication to guarantee to "hand the med, watch it fed, won't leave until it's fully swallowed"; or they sprayed insecticides in every household, immersed residents' nets house by house; or they mobilized the masses to launch the Patriotic Public Health Campaign, to fill up stagnant water pits, dredge ditches and eradicate mosquito breeding sites. As locals, barefoot doctors lived among the masses, maintaining close contact with them. Despite the low compensation for their services, the masses could afford, need, and retain their presence, and they could have easy access to nearby medical care. Even in the most remote regions, their existence guaranteed the coverage of malaria prevention and control efforts.

The barefoot doctor model in China is applicable to regions with severe shortages of health resources, providing basic health human resources and services for the poor population, which is similar to the recruitment of community health service volunteers in some African regions. Both can launch case screening, case reporting, medication treatment, insecticide mosquito killing, and environmental health management in malaria prevention and control. This model tremendously reduced costs, providing timely treatment for the poor, and are a beneficial attempt to address the basic medical care problems in poor regions of developing countries.

我国疟疾控制规划实施过程中，特别是在控制严重流行时期，在实施集体服药、灭蚊活动时，以赤脚医生为主组织服药或灭蚊小组，他们或拿药提水，挨门逐户、深入田间地头，为每个服药对象"送药到手，看服到口，不咽不走"；或深入每间房屋喷洒杀虫剂，或逐户浸泡居民蚊帐；或发动群众开展爱国卫生运动，填平积水坑洼，疏通沟渠，清除蚊虫滋生地。作为当地人，赤脚医生生活在群众之中，与群众保持密切联系，而且服务报酬不高，群众养得起、用得着、留得住，就近就医，十分方便。即使在最边远地区也有他们的存在，这就保证了抗疟工作的覆盖面。

中国的赤脚医生模式适用于卫生资源严重不足的地区，可为贫困人口提供基本卫生人力和基本卫生服务，这与非洲部分地区招募的社区卫生服务志愿者相似。在疟疾防控中都能够开展病例筛查、病例报告、服药治疗、杀虫灭蚊和环境卫生治理等工作，且提供的卫生服务都大大降低了费用，为贫困人口提供了及时的治疗，是解决发展中国家贫困地区基本医疗保健问题的一种有益的尝试。

小提示

1. 赤脚医生的优势

（1）相对于正式的医生来说，赤脚医生不需要太高深的医学知识，简单培训即可开展疟疾防治相关的诊断、治疗、报告等工作。

（2）他们可以解决农村和偏远地区缺医少药的问题，满足实际需要。

2. 赤脚医生的可行性

非洲各国的社区卫生服务人员（CHWs）就具有我国赤脚医生相类似的作用和角色：参与当地社区的临床服务、健康教育等，在疟疾防治工作中参与发现病例、RDT 快速诊断病例、给予口服抗疟药治疗、疫情报告和参与疫点调查与处置等工作。

Tips

1. Advantages of barefoot doctors

(1) Compared to formal doctors, barefoot doctors require minimal advanced medical knowledge and can make malaria prevention-related diagnosis, treatment, and carry out reporting work after simple training;

(2) They can address the problem of insufficient medical resources in rural and remote regions and meet the actual needs.

2. Feasibility of barefoot doctors

Community health workers (CHWs) in African countries have roles and functions similar to those of barefoot doctors in China: engaging in local clinical services, health education, and engaging in case detection, RDT rapid diagnosis, oral malaria treatment, endemic reporting, and engaging in endemic investigation and disposal.

3. Promotion of barefoot doctors

During the investigation in Tanzania and Zambia, it was learned that local communities needed a large number of community health service workers (or volunteers) to assist in malaria prevention and control at the grass-roots level. Regular training on malaria prevention knowledge and skills, provision of feasible means of transportation (such as bicycles), and communication tools suitable for local conditions (e.g., endemic reporting mobile phones) are necessary for local community health service personnel to provide better malaria prevention and control services.

📖 Extended Reading

Thoughts on Grass-roots Doctors in Developing Countries

In regions with large populations and underdeveloped conditions, medical resources have long been considered as a scarce resource. The barefoot doctor model in China was a proven solution to this problem during its time. In developing countries, particularly those with high disease burden and limited resources, it is crucial to draw from the excellent practices and valuable experiences of the barefoot doctor. Efforts should be made to create an environment where rural doctors can thrive, develop, and receive support. This approach should serve as an important reference for the medical systems in developing countries. Definitely, each country has its own local settings, and it is necessary to learn from experiences that have been tested by its own system and soil. Based on national conditions, continuing historical wisdom, and addressing social medical resource issues, we should create a barefoot doctor system in the new era that can adapt to local social and economic development.

3.赤脚医生的推广

从对坦桑尼亚和赞比亚的调研中发现，当地需要大量的社区卫生服务人员（或志愿者）帮助开展基层的疟疾疫情防控，需要给予当地的社区卫生服务人员定期的疟疾防治知识和技能培训，提供可行的交通工具（如自行车），符合当地条件的疫情报告通信工具（如疫情报告手机）等，以便更好地开展疟疾防控服务。

📖 拓展阅读

对发展中国家基层医生的思考

在人口众多的不发达地区，医疗资源向来稀缺，而当年中国的"赤脚医生"制度是当年解决稀缺资源的良策。而在发展中国家，特别是疾病高度流行的国家或地区，如何汲取赤脚医生制度中的优秀做法和宝贵经验，创造条件让乡村医生们留得住、能发展、有保障，应当是当今发展中国家医疗体制中值得借鉴的重要内容。当然，一国有一国之国情，借鉴那些经过自己制度和土壤检验过的经验分外必要。立足国情，延续历史智慧，解决社会医疗资源问题，我们要创造与当地社会经济发展相适应的新时代的"赤脚医生"制度。

4　Prevention and Control in Endemic Regions

4.1　Alert: Traveling to Malaria-Endemic Regions — Tips for International Travelers

Many international travelers do not properly understand malaria transmission and its personal prevention measures. They are unable to recognize the symptoms of malaria at the time of onset and often do not seek medical attention when experiencing fever or other symptoms. Besides, their lack of self-protection awareness is a major reason for malaria infection and delayed treatment.

Tips

Before travelling to tropical countries: Receive training on malaria prevention and bring antimalarial drugs.

During travelling: Utilize mosquito repellent liquids at night, wear long-sleeved clothes and long pants when going outside, and apply mosquito repellents to exposed skin.

Upon returning: Declare health status.

After returning: Seek medical attention promptly if experiencing symptoms such as fever, chills, and headache within one month.

It is recommended to undergo systematic training on malaria prevention before departure to understand what malaria is, which countries and regions it prevails in, the incubation period, and clinical manifestations after infection with different types of malaria. Travelers entering malaria endemic countries should take preventive medication, and select different doses depending upon the endemic region. Travelers should carry mosquito repellents such as floral water and wind medicated oil, using them to exposed skin like arms, neck, and calves, which are generally effective for 4 hours before reapplication. Moreover, pay attention to any allergic reactions. The efficacy of the medication is related to physical activity and sweat production. If outdoors, the duration of efficacy may be reduced, and timely reapplication is necessary. It is recommended that travelers in malaria endemic

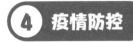

疫情防控

4.1　去有疟疾流行的地方要注意了——对国际旅行者的建议

不少国际旅行者没有正确认识疟疾和个人预防的重要性，无法有效识别疟疾发病时的症状，在有发热等症状出现的时候很多人没有就医意识，并且其自我保护意识较为薄弱，这是感染疟疾、延误治疗的主要原因。

> **小提示**
>
> 出国前：接受防疟培训，携带抗疟药品。
>
> 在国外：夜晚使用蚊香液，外出长袖和长裤，暴露皮肤用驱蚊剂。
>
> 回国时：申报健康状况。
>
> 回国后：1 个月内，若出现发热、发冷、头疼等症状，及时就诊。

建议在出国前接受系统的防疟知识培训，了解什么是疟疾，疟疾流行于哪些国家和地区，疟疾的潜伏期有多长，感染不同类型的疟疾后有哪些临床表现等。进入疟疾高发国家的旅行者应采用预防性服药，根据流行地区的不同，选择不同剂量的抗疟药物。旅行者要随身携带蚊虫驱避剂，如花露水、风油精等，一般涂抹于裸露的皮肤处，如手臂、脸颈、小腿等，一般 4 小时内有效，过了这个时间就应该重新涂抹。另外，要注意看自己是否有过敏现象。蚊虫驱避剂的药效与活动量、出汗量有关，如果在户外，药效持续时间可能会缩短，应及时补涂。建议旅行者在有疟疾流行的国家或地区，或在蚊虫活动季节，睡前在卧室喷洒杀虫剂或点蚊香，睡觉时使用蚊帐或使用拟除虫菊酯等处理的长效蚊帐，野外活动时穿长衣、长裤，皮肤暴露处可涂抹驱蚊剂，尽量避免蚊虫叮咬。旅行回国入境时，若出现发热、发冷、头疼等症

countries or during mosquito activity seasons should spray insecticides or burn mosquito coils in their bedrooms before going to sleep, use nets while sleeping, or use long-lasting nets treated with insecticides such as pyrethroids. When engaging in outdoor activities, wear long-sleeved clothes and long pants, apply mosquito repellents to exposed skin, and avoid mosquito bites as much as possible. Upon returning home, if experiencing fever, chills, and headache, actively report to port inspection and quarantine personnel to receive timely treatment. Within one month after returning, if experiencing fever, chills, and headache, promptly visit hospital and inform the medical staff of your travel history to help the diagnosis of malaria properly.

4.2　Case 7　Health Intervention for International Travelers

In recent years, the number of international travelers and participants in international exchange activities has increased because of the development of the global economy and the advancement of global integration under the Belt and Road Initiative, leading to a high incidence of imported malaria.

Once , a male patient, aged 47, who traveled to Angola in Africa on October 30, 2016, and returned about half a month later. During his stay abroad, he was once bitten by mosquitoes. On January 10, 2017, he began to get a fever with a maximum temperature of 38.7° C, but he did not seek medical care for personal reasons. On January 13 at around 17：00, the patient went to a community health center for treatment and complained of poor appetite and weakness, with a temperature of 36.7° C. He was given symptomatic treatment (anti-inflammatory and antipyretic) but showed no improvement. At 19：00, he arrived at the emergency department of a city hospital, with his family reporting slow responses for two days, unclear speech, nausea, and excessive oral secretions. On physical examination, the patient's limbs were unable to move, showing avoidance reactions upon stimulation; the pupils were 3mm on the left and 3mm on the right; a CT scan of head revealed lacunar cerebral infarction in the left basal ganglia region. The patient was diagnosed with cerebral infarction, hysteria, and malaria. After referral, laboratory tests detected *Plasmodium falciparum*, and the patient was diagnosed with falciparum malaria. On January 14, he received oral tracheal intubation and assisted ventilation, with unconsciousness and unresponsiveness to calls. Due to the severe condition and life-threatening situation, he was urgently

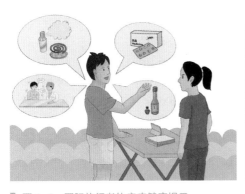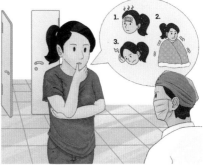

图 4-1　国际旅行者的疟疾健康提示
Figure 4-1　Malaria-Related Health Tips for International Travelers

状，应主动向口岸检验检疫人员申报，以便及时接受救治。回国后一个月内，若出现发热、发冷、头疼等症状，应当及时到医院就诊，告知医护人员自己的出入史，便于医护人员排查疟疾。

4.2　案例 7　对国际旅行者的健康干预

近年来，随着全球经济的发展以及"一带一路"倡议下全球一体化进程的推进，国际旅游及参与国际交流活动的人员日益增多，致使输入性疟疾疫情居高不下。

曾有这样一个患者，男，47 岁，于 2016 年 10 月 30 日赴非洲安哥拉境外旅游，半个月后返回，在境外居留期间曾被蚊虫叮咬。2017 年 1 月 10 日自感发热，最高体温 38.7℃，但因个人原因未及时就医。1 月 13 日 17：00 时左右患者到某社区卫生院就诊，自述食欲不佳，无力，体温 36.7℃。给予（抗炎退热）对症治疗，无好转。19：00 时转至市医院急诊，家属主诉：患者反应迟缓 2 天，言语不清、恶心、口中分泌物多。查体四肢不能活动，刺激四肢可见躲避反应，瞳孔左侧 3mm、右侧 3mm，头颅 CT 提示左基底节区腔隙性脑梗死，诊断为脑梗死、癔症、疟疾。后经转诊，化验检测查见恶性疟原

admitted to the ICU for treatment. After being admitted to the ICU, the patient was given oral tracheal intubation, mechanical ventilation, antibiotics such as piperacillin, tazobactam, and meropenem, medications to maintain organ function, and supportive treatment such as norepinephrine and continuous blood purification. He received a total of five doses of artesunate, an anti-malaria drug, at 120mg each, with the first injection at 9：20 on January 14, followed by injections every 12 hours thereafter, and the fifth injection at 9：20 on January 16. At 18：55 on January 16, the patient experienced unmeasurable blood pressure, absence of spontaneous respiration, and dilated pupils. Despite resuscitation efforts, he passed away at 19：30 on January 16 due to severe falciparum malaria (cerebral malaria) and multiple organ failure.

This falciparum malaria patient was a traveler returned from Africa who claimed never had malaria during his stay abroad. Due to a lack of awareness in prevention of malaria, the patient did not take preventive medication before or during his stay abroad. Upon returning home with fever, he did not pay enough attention and did not seek medical attention promptly for personal reasons. It was not until the fourth day of first onset that he visited a doctor. At the community health center, the patient received only general treatment for common infections. Subsequently, his condition rapidly worsened, reaching a critical state. The patient initially visited a grassroots health care facility before being referred to a higher-level medical institution. From the initial diagnosis to the confirmation of malaria, the patient visited five health facilities, and by the fifth day of illness, he had developed severe malaria, which caused the delay of the optimal diagnosis and treatment, resulting in his death.

Weak awareness of seeking medical attention and delays in seeking care are hazardous for severe malaria, which may result in unnecessary deaths. Thus, it is crucial to provide health interventions for international travelers and raise awareness of malaria diagnosis and treatment among them.

Firstly, work and rest time intervention: Provide corresponding recommendations for travelers' itineraries and destinations to avoid outdoor activities during peak mosquito activity hours. If outdoor activities are unavoidable, wear long-sleeved clothes and long pants, apply mosquito repellent to exposed skin, and avoid being bitten by mosquitoes as much as possible.

Secondly, strengthen wellness through physical exercises: Provide appropriate recommendations and guidance based on travelers' means of transportation and job nature. For instance, for those who need to work long hours at a desk,

虫，诊断为恶性疟。1月14日他接受口咽通气道辅助通气，意识不清，呼之不应。考虑病情危重，有生命危险，急收入院 ICU 治疗。入 ICU 后给予经口气管插管、呼吸机辅助机械通气，哌拉西林、他唑巴坦、美罗培南等抗生素，维护脏器的药物，以及去甲肾上腺素、连续性血液净化等支持治疗。抗疟药青蒿琥酯注射剂共用药 5 次，每次注射 120mg，1月14日9：20 第一次注射，其后每隔 12 小时注射一次，16日9：20 第五次注射。1月16日18：55，患者出现血压测不到状况，无自主呼吸，双侧瞳孔散大现象。经抢救无效于1月16日19：30 死亡。死亡原因为重症恶性疟（脑型疟）与多器官功能衰竭。

该恶性疟患者为非洲旅游归国人员，自述在国外期间未曾患有疟疾。自我防护疟疾意识不强，患者出境前和境外居留期间未服用预防药，归国出现发热症状时不重视，因个人原因未能及时就医，初次发病后第 4 天才就诊。到社区卫生院就医时仅按普通感染等进行一般治疗，而后病情进展迅速，病情危重。该患者先到基层医疗机构初诊，再转诊至上级医疗机构，从初诊到确诊辗转了 5 家医疗机构，发病第 5 天确诊时已发展为重症疟疾，耽误了最佳诊断治疗时间，致使死亡。

就诊意识弱、延误就诊是重症疟疾的危险因素之一，可能造成患者不必要的死亡。因此对国际旅行者进行健康干预，提高人群的疟疾求诊意识极其重要。

首先，作息时间干预：针对旅行者的出行计划及出行地点给出相应的建议，使旅行者尽量不在蚊虫活动高峰期到野外活动。如必须在户外，可穿长衣、长裤，皮肤暴露处可涂抹驱蚊剂，尽量避免蚊虫叮咬。

其次，运动干预：根据旅行者出行的目的，适当地给予运动建议及指导。例如，保持适度运动，避免过度疲劳以保持免疫系统的正常运作。使身心放松，更好地为其旅行做准备。

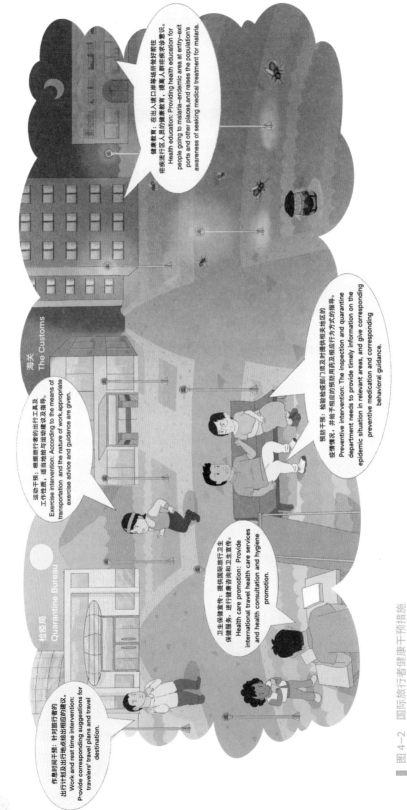

图 4-2 国际旅行者健康干预措施
Figure 4-2 Health Intervention Measures for International Travelers

1" />

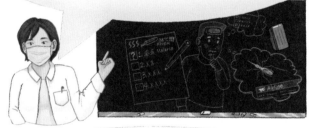

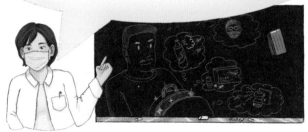

疟疾能在地球上消失吗？

099

图 4-3　给前往疟疾流行区人员的防护提示
Figure 4-3　Protection Tips for Travelers Going to Malaria-Endemic Regions

recommendations need to give them on doing do neck exercises, eye exercises, and distant gazing, etc. to relax both physically and mentally every hour, thus better preparing for their travel experience.

Thirdly, preventive measures: Due to travelers' lack of understanding of malaria, they might unknowingly visit regions where malaria is prevalent. Thus, inspection and quarantine departments need to provide timely updates on endemic situations in relevant regions and give corresponding preventive medication and behavioral guidance to effectively protect travelers' health and safety.

Fourthly, health education and promotion: Providing health care services for international travel is essential in inspection and quarantine work. Giving health consultations and conducting health promotions for incoming and outgoing travelers is also a significant responsibility. Many people are not well-informed about foreign customs and endemics. In such cases, inspection and quarantine departments need to offer all sorts of health knowledge and protection measures from a travel health perspective to enhance travelers' awareness of disease prevention abroad.

Fifthly, health education: Customs (entry-exit inspection and quarantine) should conduct health education for travelers heading to malaria-endemic regions at entry-exit ports and other locations. This will raise awareness of malaria diagnosis and remind travelers to pay attention to personal protection during their staying in malaria-endemic regions abroad. Upon returning home, travelers should seek medical attention promptly if they experience fever or other uncomfortable symptoms, actively inform medical staff about their residential history in malaria-endemic regions abroad and receive malaria screening as soon as possible. In a word, international travelers should be aware of the endemic situations and symptoms of relevant diseases in the regions they are visiting and develop effective disease prevention strategies to prepare for any contingencies depending upon their actual conditions.

4.3　Recommendations for Medical Consultation in Case of Fever in Malaria-Endemic Regions

For personnel who are preparing to travel, work, or visit malaria-endemic regions, Dr. Wang proposes the following recommendations and precautions:

(1) Determine if the destination is a malaria-endemic region. Malaria is one of the major causes of fever and severe diseases in returning travelers. Research

第三，预防干预：由于旅行者缺乏对疟疾的了解，有可能在不知情的情况下前往某些疟疾流行地区。因此，检验检疫部门须及时提供相关地区的疫情情况，并给予相应的预防用药及相应行为方式的指导，从而有效地保护旅行者的健康与安全。

第四，卫生保健宣传：提供国际旅行卫生保健服务是卫生检疫的一项重要工作，对出入境旅行人员进行健康咨询和卫生宣传也是一项重要任务。许多人对异国风情、疫情不甚了解，如对异国的水土不服，出现腹泻，这就需要检验检疫部门从旅行健康的角度向游客提供各种防病知识和保健措施，提高游客在境外的防病意识。

第五，健康教育：海关（出入境检验检疫）在出入境口岸等场所做好前往疟疾流行区人员的健康教育工作，提高人群的疟疾求诊意识，使其在国外疟疾流行区逗留期间注意个人防护，归国后出现发热等不适症状要及时就医，并主动告诉医务人员其境外疟疾流行区居留史，第一时间进行疟疾筛查。总之，国际旅行者应了解出行相关地区的疫情情况及相关疾病的发病症状，结合自身实际制定一套行之有效的防病策略，做到有备无患。

4.3 流行区发热就诊的建议

对于准备去疟疾流行地区旅行、工作、出差的人员，王医生提出以下几点建议和提示。

（1）首先要了解前往的地方是不是疟疾流行区。疟疾是旅行返回者出现发热和严重疾病的重要原因之一。研究发现，从撒哈拉以南的非洲地区返回的旅行者发生疟疾的相对风险比从亚洲或美洲返回的旅行者更高。

（2）对于去过疟疾流行区且出现发热的应首先怀疑是否感染疟疾，或者说首先要排除疟疾。非疟疾流行区的旅行者一般无免疫力，在疟疾流行区旅

has shown that travelers returning from sub-Saharan Africa have a higher risk of contracting malaria than those returning from Asia or America.

(2) For those who have visited malaria-endemic regions and developed a fever, it is advisable to consider malaria as a potential cause and seek proper diagnosis. Travelers from non-malaria-endemic regions generally have no immunity and are more susceptible to malaria infection while touring, conducting business, or working in malaria-endemic regions. Thus, malaria should be considered for patients with a fever who have a travel history in malaria-endemic regions. Their chances of developing severe malaria are high after contracting falciparum malaria.

(3) Take personal protection measures when visiting malaria-endemic regions. Travelers to malaria transmission regions should be aware of the risks they might face, as these regions pose a severe infection that can be fatal within just a few days. Precautions include avoiding mosquito bites and adhering to malaria chemoprophylaxis. However, travelers should also be aware that no chemical prophylaxis can provide 100% protection, and any fever occurring during or after the journey is a medical emergency that requires immediate consultation.

4.4 Why Should Disease Management in Border Regions be Strengthened?

Tips

In tropical and subtropical border regions, cross-border movements of people, mosquitoes, and goods can cause cross-border transmission of malaria, making malaria prevention and control and elimination in border regions extremely challenging. In Yunnan Province of China, a long-term malaria prevention and control campaign has led to the implementation of the "3 + 1" strategy, achieving the goal of malaria elimination and preventing reestablishment in border regions.

4.4.1 Channels of Imported Malaria Cases

Tips

Malaria cases are generally imported through three channels: personnel from malaria-endemic regions, overseas returnees from non-malaria-endemic regions, and *Anopheles* mosquitoes.

游、经商、工作时更容易感染疟疾。因此，对于有疟区旅行史的发热患者，均应考虑疟疾。他们在感染恶性疟后极可能导致重症疟疾发生。

（3）前往疟疾流行区要做好个人防护。前往疟疾传播地区的旅行者应了解其面临的疟疾感染风险，这是一种仅需数日病程即可致命的严重感染。预防措施包括避免蚊虫叮咬和坚持抗疟疾化学预防等。然而，旅行者也应该了解到，没有任何一种化学预防方案可以百分百做到完全防护，旅程中或返回后出现发热是医疗急症，需要紧急就诊。

4.4　为什么要加强边境地区的疾病管理？

小提示

在热带和亚热带边境地区，人、蚊虫和货物跨境流动均会引起疟疾跨境传播，致使边境疟疾控制和消除极为困难。我国云南省在长期边境疟疾防控中，总结出了"3+1"策略，实现了在边境地区消除疟疾和防止输入再传播的目标。

4.4.1　疟疾输入渠道

小提示

疟疾一般通过来自疟区人员、非疟区出境回归人员和按蚊三种方式输入。

为防止疟疾输入再传播，首先需要了解疟疾输入非流行区的三种渠道：①通过来自疟疾流行国家或地区（疟区）人员携带疟原虫的输入；②非疟区人员出境到疟区，感染疟疾回归后的输入；③疟区感染疟原虫蚊虫（按蚊）进入非疟区引起疟疾传播的输入。

第三种输入渠道中，宽体飞机携带感染疟原虫按蚊在机场及附近引起传播的疟疾，叫机场疟疾；轮船携带感染疟原虫按蚊在港口及附近引起传播的

To prevent malaria importation and reestablishment, it is first necessary to understand the three channels of malaria imported cases into non-endemic regions: ① Imported through malaria parasites carried by personnel from malaria endemic countries or regions (malaria-endemic regions); ② Imported through people migrated from non-malaria-endemic regions to malaria-endemic regions and get malaria; ③ Imported cases caused by *Anopheles* mosquitoes infected with malaria parasites from malaria-endemic regions to non-malaria-endemic regions.

In the third transmission channel, *Anopheles* mosquitoes can be transported by wide-body aircraft, causing malaria to spread at airports and nearby regions, which is referred to as airport malaria. Similarly, ships carry *Anopheles* mosquitoes infected with malaria parasites, causing malaria to spread in ports and nearby regions, which is called port malaria. Malaria transmitted by *Anopheles* mosquitoes imported from malaria-bordering regions into non-malaria border regions is known as malaria spilled from overseas borders.

Non-malaria border regions can simultaneously have these three transmission channels, with malaria spill over from overseas borders being closely related to the flying distance of *Anopheles* mosquitoes. Global data from experiments on nearly 300 *Anopheles* mosquitoes marked and released show that under normal circumstances, the flying distance of *Anopheles* mosquitoes does not exceed 2.5 kilometers, usually within 1 kilometer. Regions within 1 kilometer of non-malaria border regions are severely affected by malaria imported from overseas borders, and imported malaria increases with proximity to malaria-endemic regions.

4.4.2　The "3 + 1" Strategy for Preventing Malaria Re-Establishment

In response to the problem of simultaneous existence of three malaria transmission channels in border regions, the Yunnan border region adopts the "3 + 1" management strategy to prevent malaria import and re-establishment.

"1" : Implement comprehensive preventive measures that focus on both sources of disease transmission and vector surveillance in villages within 2.5 kilometers of the border to address the issue of frequent cross-border movement of people and the spread of malaria caused by *Anopheles* mosquitoes crossing the border. Specific measures include: ① Promptly identifying imported malaria cases through passive and active surveillance of infection sources, conducting standardized treatment and disease control measures, and blocking transmission in a timely manner; ② Strengthening the surveillance of *Anopheles* mosquitoes as vectors, using indoor residual spraying of insecticides and other vector control

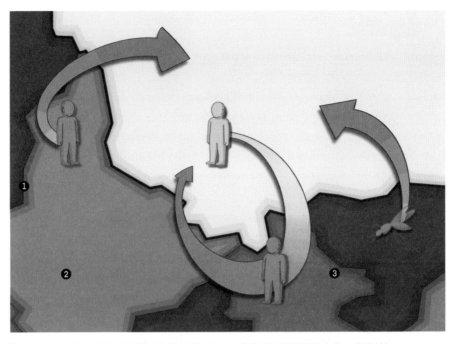

图 4-4　三种疟疾输入渠道（①来自疟区人员；②非疟区出境回归人员；③按蚊）
Figure 4-4　Three Malaria Transmission Channels（① personnel from malaria-endemic regions；② returnees from non-malaria-endemic regions；③ *Anopheles* mosquitoes）

疟疾，称港口疟疾；来自疟区边境地区携带疟原虫按蚊飞越边界进入非疟区边境地区引起传播的疟疾，称境外边境外溢疟疾。

非疟区的边境地区可同时存在这 3 种疟疾输入渠道，其中境外边境外溢疟疾与按蚊飞行距离紧密相关。全球近 300 只按蚊标记放飞试验结果显示，正常情况下，按蚊飞行距离不超过 2.5 公里，一般在 1 公里内。非疟区距离境外疟区 1 公里范围内的地区，是受境外边境外溢疟疾影响最严重的地区，而且距离境外疟疾流行社区越近，感染境外边境外溢疟疾的风险越高。

4.4.2　防止疟疾输入再传播"3+1"策略

针对边境地区同时存在三种疟疾输入渠道的问题，云南边境地区采用"3+1"管理策略，防止疟疾输入再传播。

症
疾
能
在
地
球
上
消
失
吗
？

The focus of the "3 + 1" strategy is to adopt comprehensive prevention and control measures within the flying distance of *Anopheles* mosquitoes, reducing malaria import caused by positive *Anopheles* mosquitoes (1); timely discovering malaria import from frequent cross-border people, especially those who enter from informal ports, in front-line towns and villages (2); comprehensively strengthening the border counties' malaria surveillance and rapid response system with "health facilities as the main body and CDC as the center" to timely prevent malaria import and re-transmission (3); and enhancing cooperation with neighboring countries in malaria control in border regions to reduce the transmission level and malaria importation (+ 1).

measures when the density of vector *Anopheles* mosquitoes is high, thereby lowering the risk of malaria being imported from overseas; ③ Implementing additional preventive drugs to protect the border residents when the malaria endemic level and the density of *Anopheles* mosquitoes abroad are too high, and the domestic vector control measures are insufficient to effectively reduce the importation of malaria from overseas; ④ Enhancing health education to improve the personal protection capacities of border residents.

"2" : Adopting a community-based strategy to strengthen the surveillance of sources of infection for the first-line villages in border towns and villages, where relatives and friends of the same ethnic group live across borders, and there are complex situations such as "one village cross two countries" and "cross-border marriage" , resulting in increased risk of malaria importation due to frequent cross-border movement of people. Taking passive and active detection measures to find malaria patients. Apart from the malaria tests conducted by the township health center, village cadres and villagers should assist in referring incoming fever patients to the township health center for malaria testing through effective communication and coordination. In remote villages where it takes more than an hour to walk to the health center or half an hour to ride a motorcycle, training village health workers or malaria prevention personnel to use rapid diagnostic kits to detect malaria. When suspicious clues of imported malaria cases are detected, promptly report to the county disease control center for investigation and response. Meanwhile, strengthen health education to enhance the prevention awareness and self-protection capabilities of local residents and cross-border personnel, as well as to

"3+1"策略的工作重点是，在按蚊飞行距离内采用综合性防控措施，减少阳性按蚊引起的疟疾输入（1）；在边境一线乡镇及时发现频繁跨境人员，特别是从非正式口岸入境人员的疟疾输入（2）；全面加强边境县以"医疗机构为主，以 CDC 为中心"的疟疾监测和快速响应体系，及时发现疟疾，防止输入再传播（3）；加强与邻国边境地区的疟疾防控合作以降低其流行程度，减少输入（+1）。

"1"：在距离边境线 2.5 公里范围内的村寨，采取传染源和媒介监测并重的综合预防措施，以解决人员频繁跨境流动，按蚊飞越国际边界引发境外边境外溢疟疾的问题。具体措施包括：①通过传染源的被动和主动侦查，及时发现输入疟疾病例，进行规范治疗和疫情处置，及时阻断传播；②加强媒介按蚊监测，发现媒介按蚊密度较高时，采用杀虫剂室内滞留喷洒等媒介控制措施降低按蚊密度，从而降低境外边境外溢疟疾风险；③当境外疟疾流行程度和按蚊密度过高，境内的媒介控制措施又不足以有效减少境外边境外溢疟疾时，增加预防服药措施保护边境居民；④加强健康教育，增强边民个人防护能力。

"2"：针对边境乡镇一线村寨，同一民族的亲朋好友跨境而居，存在"一寨两国"和"跨境婚姻"等复杂情况，人员的频繁跨境流动导致疟疾输入风险增高，采用以社区为基础的策略加强传染源监测。采取被动和主动侦查并重措施发现疟疾患者，除乡镇卫生院开展疟疾检测外，通过有效沟通交流，村干部和村民应协助推介入境发热患者到乡镇卫生院接受疟疾检测。在步行到卫生院需要 1 小时以上，或骑摩托需要半小时以上的边远村寨，培训村卫生员或疟防员使用快速诊断试剂盒检测疟疾，发现输入性疟疾可疑线索时，及时通知县疾控中心进行调查和处理。同时，加强健康教育，增强当地居民和跨境人员的疟疾预防意识和自我保护能力，提高边境社区居民推介入境发热患者到乡镇卫生院接受疟疾检测的意识。

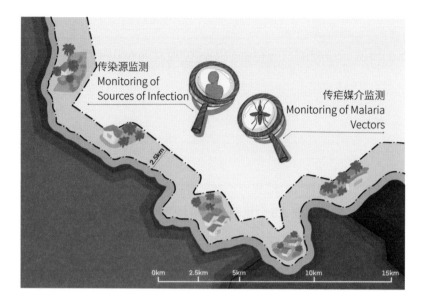

1：在距境外社区 2.5 千米范围内加强传染源和媒介监测及综合防治措施
1: Strengthen the monitoring of infectious sources and vectors and comprehensive prevention and control measures within 2.5km of overseas communities

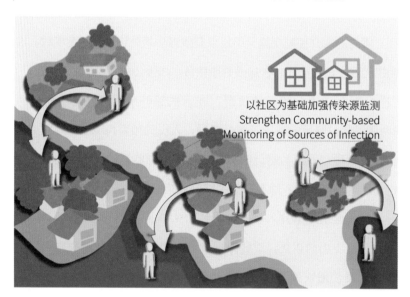

2：在边境一线乡镇，动员群众参与，及时发现输入疟疾
2: Mobilize the residents in the border villages and townships for timely detection of imported malaria

图 4-5 边境疟疾"3+1"防控策略
Figure 4-5 "3 + 1" Prevention and Control Strategy of Malaria in Border Regions

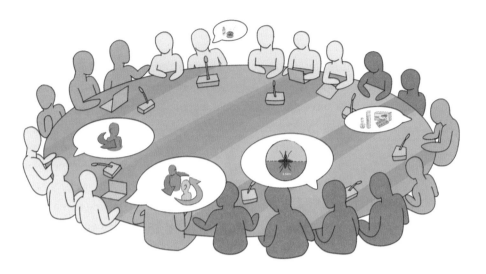

3：在边境区县加强以医疗卫生机构为主的疟疾检测和监测体系建设
3: Strengthen the building of malaria diagnosis and surveillance systems led by medical and health institutions in border areas and counties

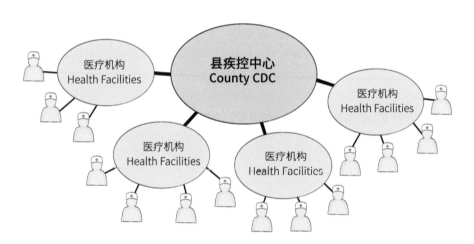

+1：加强与邻国的合作，降低其边境地区疟疾流行程度以减少输入
+1: Strengthen cooperation with neighboring countries to reduce malaria prevalence in their border areas to reduce malaria importation

raise the referral consciousness of incoming fever patients to the township health center among border community residents.

"3" : To guarantee timely detection of imported malaria, standardized treatment and the elimination of the sources of infection, strengthen the construction of malaria surveillance and rapid response system based on "health facilities" and dominated by "county CDC" in border counties. After discovering imported malaria cases, the county CDC should review, investigate, and respond to control of malaria re-transmission in line with the "1-3-7" norm. This includes involving all medical and health facilities (including pharmacies) in malaria case detection through effective communication; annually providing training to maintain health personnel, particularly clinical doctors' malaria knowledge and alertness to imported malaria cases; and promoting multi-sectoral cooperation, health education, and timely referral of returning fever patients to health facilities with malaria testing capacities.

"+ 1" : Sharing malaria prevention and control technology and information, improving prevention and control capabilities for imported malaria cases from overseas borders, jointly dealing with sudden malaria outbreaks in cross-border regions, reducing the prevalence of malaria abroad, and lowering the risks of domestic malaria re-transmission by strengthening joint prevention and control cooperation on malaria cases imported from overseas borders.

4.5 Case 8 Model of Regional Cooperation: Joint Prevention and Control of Malaria in Five Provinces

Tips

The prevalence of malaria requires certain natural climatic and human conditions. Within a certain regional scope, the natural climate and human characteristics are roughly similar, and the prevalence of diseases is also the same. When an outbreak occurred, unified actions need to be taken across the entire region to respond, which is known as regional cooperation mechanism for joint prevention and control of malaria.

During a malaria outbreak, the endemic may cross village, township, even provincial and international boundaries due to the activities of patients and mosquitoes. In the process of controlling malaria prevalence, a joint prevention

"3"：为确保能及时发现输入疟疾和规范治疗，清除传染源，加强边境县"以医疗机构为基础，以县疾控中心为主"的疟疾监测和快速响应体系建设。发现输入疟疾病例后，县疾控中心应按"1-3-7"工作规范复核、调查和处理。包括通过有效交流沟通，让全体医疗卫生机构（包括药店）参与疟疾病例的检测；每年通过培训，维持卫生人员，特别是临床医生的疟疾知识和对输入疟疾的警觉性；通过多部门合作、开展健康教育、促进境外回归发热患者及时到有疟疾检查能力的医疗卫生机构求医。

"+1"：通过加强跨境疟疾联防联控合作，共享疟疾防控技术和信息，提高境外疟疾防控能力，共同处理境外边境地区疟疾突发疫情，降低境外疟疾流行程度，减少来自境外的输入性疟疾，降低境内疟疾再传播的风险。

4.5 案例8 区域合作的典范：五省疟疾联防联控

小提示

　　疟疾的流行需要一定的自然气候和人文条件，而在一定的区域范围内，自然气候和人文特征大致相似，疾病的流行程度也相仿，当有疫情发生时，需要在整个区域内采取统一的行动来应对，这就是区域联防联控。

当发生疟疾流行时，由于患者及蚊子的活动，疫情可能跨越村与村的边界、乡与乡的边界，甚至省与省的边界和国与国的边界。在控制疟疾流行过程中，我国创立了具有中国特色的疟区联防联控机制。实践证明，建立疟疾区域性联防，有利于争取各级领导的支持，有利于互相交流与促进，有利于发动群众，有利于各项抗疟措施的落实，是加快疟疾防控步伐，巩固和扩大抗疟成果的一种有效方法。

and control mechanism for malaria-endemic regions with Chinese characteristics was created. Practices have proven that establishing regional joint prevention and control of malaria is beneficial to securing support from all levels of leadership, promoting mutual exchange and promotion, mobilizing the masses, and implementing all types of malaria prevention and control measures, which is an effective method to accelerate the pace of malaria prevention and control, consolidate and expand malaria prevention and control achievements.

1. What is the joint prevention and control mechanism for malaria-endemic regions?

The mechanism is a joint prevention and control system composed of different administrative regions with adjacent locations, similar natural conditions, consistent endemic factors, and similar endemic levels under the organization or guidance of higher-level governments or health authorities. Under the guidance of superior specialized technical departments, the professional technical units of malaria prevention and control in the joint prevention and control regions jointly work out malaria prevention and control strategies and measures, adopt unified plans, synchronous actions and joint training, conduct information exchanges and "grinding mill" mutual inspection, and organize regular meetings for experience sharing.

2. How was the joint prevention and control mechanism of Jiangsu, Shandong, Henan, Anhui and Hubei Provinces in China established?

In the 1960s and 1970s, the five provinces of Jiangsu, Shandong, Henan, Anhui and Hubei experienced two large-scale malaria outbreaks. In 1970, the reported cases in these five provinces (21.984 million) accounted for 91.16% of the total malaria cases reported nationwide. Despite the decrease in the number of cases after the prevention and control measures taken in 1971-1972, the reported malaria cases in the five provinces were still up to 13.7294 million in 1973. Under the guidance of the State Council and the organization of the National Health Commission, an agreement for the joint prevention and control of malaria in five provinces was signed in Zhengzhou City in December 1974 in view of the same species of malaria parasites and similar species and ecological habits of *Anopheles* mosquitoes in the five provinces. The agreement stipulated that each province would send 10 people to form five inspection teams from July 1 to 10 of each year, with the team leaders being responsible for the health bureaus of each province. The teams would implement a "grinding mill" inspection of malaria prevention and

1. 什么是疟区联防联控机制？

在上级政府或卫生主管部门的组织或指导下，由相互毗邻、自然条件相似、流行因素一致、流行程度相近的不同行政区域组成联防联控体系，在上级专业技术部门的指导下，联防地区的疟疾防控专业技术单位共同制定疟疾防控的策略和措施，统一计划，同步行动，联合培训，互通信息，"推磨式"交互检查，定期召开会议交流经验。

2. 苏鲁豫皖鄂联防联控机制是如何建立起来的？

20世纪60年代和70年代，苏鲁豫皖鄂五省曾发生两次大范围的疟疾暴发流行,1970年五省报告疟疾病例数（2 198.4万）占全国报告疟疾病例总数的91.16%。经1971年至1972年的防治，疟疾病例数虽有所减少，但1973年5省疟疾报告病例数仍高达1 372.94万。在国务院的直接指导和国家卫生部的组织下,针对五省区域内疟原虫种相同、媒介按蚊种类和生态习性相似的特点，1974年12月，五省在郑州达成了五省疟疾联防联控的协议。协议商定：每年7月1日至10日，每省10人，混编组成5个检查团，团长由各省卫生局负责同志担任，对五省疟防工作实施推磨式检查。

3. 苏鲁豫皖鄂联防联控机制取得了哪些成效？

根据传播媒介中华按蚊兼吸人畜血、偏室外吸血及野栖习性特点，位于中国中部的黄淮平原的五省组成联防联控片区，统一采取以控制传染源为主的综合防治策略，在1974年至1979年大范围暴发流行时，重点抓好传播季节全民预防服药和传播休止期全民根治服药的"两全服药"（即全民根治和全民预防服药）措施，取得了良好效果。到1979年，五省疟疾病例数降至191.41万,较1973年减少了86.06%，较1970年减少了91.29%。

1980年后五省继续实施联防，并根据疟疾流行程度及自然、社会因素的变化，调整联防的指导思想和技术措施。江苏、河南和安徽三省交界毗邻地

control in the five provinces.

3. What achievements has Jiangsu, Shandong, Henan, Anhui and Hubei joint prevention and control mechanism made?

Given the characteristics of *Anopheles sinensis*, which acts as a vector for both human and animal blood, prefers outdoor blood sucking, and is wild-residing, the five provinces in central China's Huang-Huai Plain formed a joint prevention and control area and adopted a comprehensive prevention and control strategy focused on controlling the sources of infection. During the large-scale outbreak in 1974-1979, they laid emphasis on the "two-wide medication" (i.e., nationwide radical cure before transmission season, and nationwide mess drug administration during transmission season) measures during the transmission season and the non-transmission phase, achieving good results. By 1979, the number of cases in the five provinces decreased to 1.9141 million, with a 86.06% reduction from 1973 and a 91.29% reduction from 1970.

Following the year of 1980, the five provinces continued to implement joint prevention and control measures, and adjusted the guiding principle and technical measures based on the malaria prevalence, as well as changes in natural and social factors. The border regions of Jiangsu, Henan, and Anhui provinces jointly adopted comprehensive prevention and control measures consisting of residual spraying of DDT and pyrethroid insecticide treated nets, and they respectively achieved the goal of eliminating falciparum malaria between 1988 and 1991.

After 2000, in response to the resurgence and local outbreak of vivax malaria in the northern region of the Huaihe River, the five provinces effectively controlled the rising transmission and local outbreaks through timely reporting of epidemic information, mutual exchange of prevention and control experiences, joint exploration of countermeasures, and joint strengthening of prevention and control measures. By 2008, there were up to 6,195 malaria cases annually in the five provinces, accounting for only 23.59% of the national total, and the average annual incidence rate decreased to 0.69 per 10,000.

4. What are the significant implications of the joint prevention and control system?

(1) The system is based on a common commitment to malaria prevention and control. The five provinces have all strengthened leadership in malaria prevention and control to avoid affecting other regions due to inadequate management, and actively provided support for the prevention and control.

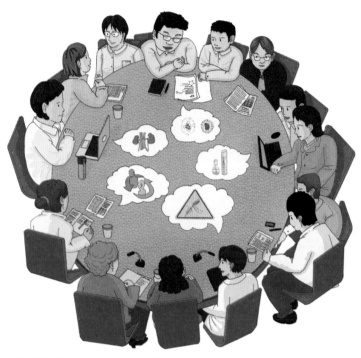

图 4-6 区域联防联控商讨对付疟疾的策略
Figure 4-6 Discuss malaria prevention and control strategies through Regional Joint Prevention and Control

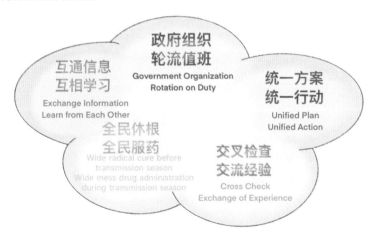

图 4-7 通过区域联防联控有利于加快疟疾防控步伐
Figure 4-7 Accelerating Malaria Control Programme Through Regional Joint Prevention and Control Mechanism

(2) The system effectively avoids the dissemination of infection sources or vectors caused by varying progress in prevention and control through implementing unified strategies and technical measures, thus contributing to the consolidation of prevention and control achievements.

(3) The system enables neighboring regions to promptly respond to outbreaks through exchanging information, taking timely interventions to prevent or curb the spread of the endemic.

(4) The system helps to identify weak the gaps within the scope of joint prevention and control through mutual inspection and exchange of experiences, jointly addressing difficulties and continuously promoting the progress of malaria control programme.

Tips

1. Advantages of Joint Defense and Control Mechanism in Five Provinces

(1) Malaria is a rapidly spreading and acute infectious disease. Hence, the prevalence and effectiveness of malaria prevention and control in adjacent regions often influence and restrict each other in the process of prevention and control. Thus, several administrative regions with adjacent locations, similar natural conditions, identical endemic factors, and similar prevalence levels should be organized based on the prevention and control needs of a certain period, to establish a regional joint prevention against malaria and jointly work out prevention and control strategies and measures, implement unified plans, synchronize actions, conduct joint training, exchange information, inspect each other, share experiences, conduct evaluations and commendations, so that the malaria prevention is both grand and practical, effectively promoting the in-depth development of malaria control programmes.

(2) Establishing a regional joint prevention against malaria is beneficial to strive for the support of leaders at all levels, promote exchanges and mutual learning, mobilize the masses, and guarantee the implementation of all types of malaria prevention and control measures. It is an effective method to accelerate the pace of malaria control programmes, consolidate and expand the achievements of anti-malaria efforts.

2. Reproducibility of the Joint Prevention and Control of the Five Provinces

(1) In 2017, in order to further consolidate the achievements of malaria elimination and prevent re-transmission caused by imported malaria, the former

区共同采取 DDT 滞留喷洒和菊酯类杀虫剂浸泡蚊帐为主的综合防治措施，并在 1988 年至 1991 年间实现了消除恶性疟的目标。

2000 年以后，五省针对沿淮河以北地区出现的间日疟疫情回升和局部暴发流行，通过即时通报疫情信息、相互交流防治经验、共同探讨防治对策和共同加强防控措施等，有效控制了疫情回升和局部的暴发流行。到 2008 年，五省疟疾发病 6 195 例，在全国发病数的占比降至 23.59%，平均年发病率降至 0.69 人次 / 万。

4. 联防联控体系的重要意义有哪些？

（1）该体系以共同承诺做好疟疾防控为基础，为避免因自我防治不力对其他地区造成影响，五省均加强了对疟防工作的领导，并积极为防控工作提供保障。

（2）通过贯彻统一的防治策略和技术措施，有效避免了由于防治工作进程不一造成的传染源或传播媒介的扩散，有利于防治成果的巩固。

（3）通过互通信息，及时了解毗邻地区的突发疫情等情况，使毗邻地区能及时采取应对措施防止或遏制疫情的蔓延。

（4）通过相互检查和经验交流，及时发现联防范围内防治工作中的薄弱环节，共同及时解决防治工作中的困难，持续推进防治工作。

小提示

1. 五省联防联控的优势

（1）疟疾是一种迅速蔓延的急性传染病，因此在防控过程中疟疾的流行程度和防治效果，在毗邻地区往往是相互影响和制约的，因而根据某个时期的防治需求，由相互毗邻、自然条件相似、流行因素相同、流行程度相近的若干行政区域组织起来，建立区域性的抗疟联防，共同制定防治策略和措施，并实行

National Health Commission developed a joint prevention and control mechanism for malaria elimination, wherein the 24 malaria-endemic provinces in the country were divided into four joint prevention and control regions to collaborate on malaria elimination.

(2) Future joint prevention and control mechanisms of malaria should not be limited to regions, but should also involve the participation of departments, e.g., health care centers of customs, business and cultural tourism departments. By 2018, 22 provinces had set up joint prevention and control mechanisms.

4.6　Recommendations for the Timeliness of Malaria Surveillance

The timeliness of infectious disease surveillance is an important indicator in the quality management of infectious disease surveillance, which refers to the process of early detection, timely reporting of infectious diseases by health facilities, and response and disposal by the disease control institutions upon the receipt of the reports. The timeliness and effectiveness of the entire process play a decisive role in the prevention of infectious diseases and the control of epidemics. In accordance with the *Law of the People's Republic of China on the Prevention and Treatment of Infectious Diseases*, infectious diseases are divided into Class A, Class B, and Class C. As a Class B infectious disease, malaria requires reporting within 24 hours after case detection.

In the past, China's infectious disease surveillance reports were compiled by disease control institutions using statistical tables, which were gradually summarized and reported up the hierarchy. However, these reports lacked timely information, were time-consuming and labor-intensive in data handling, and did not able to provide timely access to information. After 2003, the national government stressed the construction of the web-based health information platform and mechanism for the timeliness of infectious disease surveillance reports. Based on the browser/server (B/S) architecture, a national disease prevention and infectious disease surveillance system was set up, which was implemented nationwide starting from January 1, 2004. The system implemented case-based management of infectious diseases, with malaria being one of the diseases under surveillance. The timeliness of malaria transmission reporting was significantly raised.

统一计划，同步行动，联合培训，互通信息，相互检查，交流经验，评比表彰，既使得疟防工作轰轰烈烈，又能扎扎实实推动疟疾防治工作深入发展。

（2）建立疟疾区域性联防，有利于争取各级领导的支持，有利于交流和互相促进，有利于发动群众，有利于各项抗疟措施的落实，是加快疟疾防治步伐，巩固和扩大抗疟成果的一种有效方法。

2. 五省联防联控的可推广性

（1）2017 年，为进一步巩固消除疟疾成果，防止输入疟疾引起再传播，原国家卫生健康委员会制订了消除疟疾联防联控机制，将全国 24 个流行省分为 4 个联防联控区域，协作开展消除疟疾工作。

（2）未来的疟疾联防联控机制不应局限于区域，还应吸纳部门参与，如海关的卫生保健中心、商务和文旅等部门。截至 2018 年，已有 22 个省份建立了联合预防与控制机制。

4.6 疟疾监测时效性的建议

传染病监测时效性作为传染病监测质量管理的重要指标，是指医疗机构对传染病的早期发现、及时报告和疾病预防控制机构收到报告后响应处置的过程，整个过程的及时有效对传染病的预防和疫情的控制起到决定性作用。根据《中华人民共和国传染病防治法》，传染病分为甲类、乙类和丙类。疟疾作为乙类传染病，要求在病例发现后 24 小时内上报。

以往中国传染病监测报告是由疾病预防控制机构用统计表逐级汇总上报，这些报告缺少及时信息，费时、费工，且无法适时得到信息。2003 年后国家高度重视传染病监测报告时效性的平台与机制建设，建立了基于浏览器 / 服务器（B/S）构架的国家疾病预防传染病监测系统，自 2004 年 1 月 1 日起全国推行，并对传染病实行个案管理，疟疾为监测病种之一，疫情报告时效性得到全面提高。

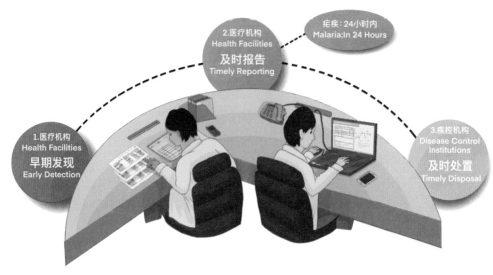

图 4-8　发现疟疾病例后及时（24 小时内）报告
Figure 4-8　Prompt reporting of malaria cases within 24 hours

4.7　Are There Prophylactic Drugs? Are They Effective?

There are several prophylactic drugs for antimalarial infections, with chloroquine phosphate or piperaquine being the preferred medications. However, no preventive drug provides a 100% protective effect against malaria infection. Prophylactic drugs must be used in consideration of the drug resistance in different regions, and anti-malaria drugs are generally taken with food and accompanied by plenty of water. Regular medication is necessary, and careful consideration should be given before use.

In mixed malaria-endemic regions of falciparum malaria and vivax malaria, one monthly dose of piperaquine phosphate, 600mg oral administration, is recommended during the transmission season. The medication should be taken before going to bed. The continuous use of medication should not exceed 4 months, and the next preventive medication should be administered at an interval of 2-3 months; in single endemic region with only vivax malaria, one dose of piperaquine phosphate, 300mg oral administration, is recommended every 7-10 days during the endemic season. The medication should be taken before going to bed. Anti-malaria drugs are generally taken with food and accompanied by plenty of water. Regular medication is necessary. Each anti-malaria preventive drug

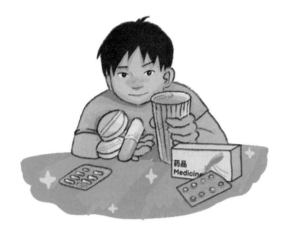

图 4-9　前往高危疫区者可提前服用疟疾预防药
Figure 4-9　People who travel to high-risk areas can take malaria prophylactic medicine

4.7　有预防药吗？服了管用吗？

疟疾有预防药，磷酸氯喹或哌喹可作首选剂。没有任何一种预防药有百分之百的保护作用，预防用药必须根据不同地区而使用不同的药物，抗疟药一般跟食物一起服用，而且要喝大量的水，服药必须规律，使用前必须仔细考虑。

在恶性疟和间日疟的混合流行地区，在流行季节每月服用磷酸哌喹一次，每次口服 600mg，临睡前服用，连续用药不超过 4 个月，再次进行预防服药应间隔 2～3 个月；在单一间日疟流行地区，在流行季节每 7～10 日服用磷酸哌喹一次，每次口服 300mg，临睡前服用。抗疟疾药物一般跟食物一起服用，而且要喝大量的水，服药必须规律。每种抗疟预防药物都有不同人群使用的禁忌，使用前必须仔细考虑。曾经前往疫区的民众必须了解，不管有无使用预防用药，回国后 1 个月内若有原因不明的发热，应尽早就医，并主动告知医师相关的旅游史。

has contraindications for different populations. Careful consideration should be given before use. It is essential for people who have traveled to endemic regions to understand that whether or not they have taken preventive medication, if they have unexplained fever within 1 months after returning to their home country, they should seek medical attention promptly and actively inform the doctor about their travel history.

4.8 Case 9 Rapid Control of Malaria Outbreaks in Central China: Mass Drug Administration

Tips

Practice is the sole criterion for testing truth. There are a variety of methods for rapidly response to the malaria outbreaks, among which mass drug administration (MDA) is undoubtedly the most effective measure in central China.

Since the 1930s, MDA has been adopted for malaria control programmes, and in the 1950s, the WHO recommended its use for controlling malaria epidemics. Currently, the WHO suggests implementing focal MDA in regions where malaria is on the verge of being eradicated, e.g., blocking the transmission of falciparum malaria and lowering the transmission risks of multi-drug resistant malaria in the Greater Mekong Region.

China once extensively used MDA to control malaria epidemics in the 1970s and 1980s, achieving significant results. Before 1949, China had approximately 30 million malaria cases on an annual basis. In 1970, the number of cases was over 24 million, with 91.2% concentrated in five provinces in the central region (including Henan, Jiangsu, Shandong, Anhui, and Hubei provinces), mainly due to vivax malaria. These five provinces jointly adopted unified comprehensive prevention and control measures centered on eliminating the sources of infection, including MDA during the transmission season and radical cure in the non-transmission season, and mass prophylactic medication during the transmission season. The MDA for radical cure in non-transmission season refers to giving all residents in malaria-endemic regions a total of 180mg of primaquine for an 8-day therapy during the annual Spring Festival in order to eradicate liver-stage delayed-type sporozoites and prevent from malaria recurrence. The mass prophylactic

4.8　案例 9　中国中部地区迅速控制疟疾疫情：大规模人群服药

小提示

　　实践是检验真理的唯一标准，迅速控制疟疾疫情的方法有多种，大规模人群服药无疑是中国中部地区最有效的措施。

　　自 20 世纪 30 年代以来，大规模人群服药一直用于疟疾控制，50 年代世卫组织曾推荐将其用于控制疟疾流行。目前世卫组织建议针对即将消除疟疾的地区，在阻断恶性疟传播和降低大湄公河区域多药耐药性疟疾传播风险等情况下实施大规模人群服药。

　　中国在 20 世纪的 70 年代和 80 年代曾广泛使用大规模人群服药控制疟疾流行并取得显著成果。1949 年以前中国每年大约有 3 000 万疟疾病例。1970 年发病人数超过 2 400 万，91.2% 集中在中部的五个省份（河南、江苏、山东、安徽和湖北），主要为间日疟。五个省联合行动、采取统一的以消灭传染源为主的综合性防治措施，其中传播休止期全民服药和传播季节全民预防服药都是大规模人群服药。传播休止期全民服药是指每年春节在疟疾传播休止期对疟疾流行严重地区的所有居民给予伯氨喹总量 180mg 的 8 日疗法以清除肝期迟发型子孢子，防止疟疾复发。传播季节全民预防服药是指在夏秋疟疾流行季节对疟疾流行严重地区的所有居民给予氯喹总量 1 200mg 加伯氨喹总量 180mg 的 8 日疗法，以清除可能的传染源。1974 年至 1979 年 5 省 3 亿人口中，4.17 亿人接受传播休止期全民服药，6.03 亿人接受传播季节全民预防服药。五个省的疟疾病例从 1973 年的 1 373 万例减少到 1979 年的 191 万例，减少了 86.06%。疟疾发病率在 10% 以上的县由 1973 年的 145 个下降到 1979 年的 15 个；发病率为 1% ～ 10% 的县数由 203 个下降到 102 个，五个省中疟疾发病率低于 1 人次 / 万的有 94 个。

medication during the transmission season refers to administering a total of 1200mg of chloroquine and 180mg of primaquine for an 8-day therapy to all residents in severely malaria-endemic regions during the high transmission season of summer and autumn in order to eliminate the potential sources of infection. From 1974 to 1979, among the 300 million people in the five provinces, 417 million individuals/times received MDA during the non-transmission for radical cure, and 603 million individuals/times received mass prophylactic medication during the transmission season. The number of malaria cases in the five provinces decreased from 13.73 million in 1973 to 1.91 million in 1979, a reduction of 86.06%. The number of counties with a malaria incidence rate of over 10% decreased from 145 in 1973 to 15 in 1979; and the number of counties with an incidence rate of 1% to 10% decreased from 203 to 102. Among the five provinces, 94 counties had a malaria incidence rate below 1/10,000.

During MDA, personnel involving in malaria control programmes frequently carried thermos bottles and medicine boxes, visiting households, fields, and various locations, implementing medication through "hand the med,watch it fed,won't leave until it's fully swallowed, and providing a replacement if vomited" . They also utilized comprehensible and catchy phrases, e.g., "Malaria is transmitted by mosquitoes, taking medicine is free, so hurry up and see the health worker if you have malaria" , widely painting them on the walls of residential buildings to guarantee that they were ubiquitous, making the public not only able to see them when they looked up but also understand and remember them, and retaining the information for a long time.

Yongcheng City, Henan Province, achieved the standard of basic malaria elimination (with an incidence rate below 1/10,000) in 1991, with no local malaria cases reported for 11 consecutive years. However, the number of malaria cases rapidly increased from 2003 to 2006; in 2006, 36 outbreaks were detected in four townships; the number of malaria cases in Yongcheng City accounted for 56.78% of the total cases in the province in 2006. From 2007 to 2009, a large-scale MDA was launched to 183,688 people in 5 townships and 91 villages of Yongcheng City. The treatment success rate of the whole course was over 96%. The malaria incidence rate plummeted, and the last local malaria case was reported in 2011. In 2018, it was confirmed that malaria had been eliminated in the city.

The process from implementation for control to elimination is a long-term and arduous task that requires prolonged and repetitive prevention and control measures

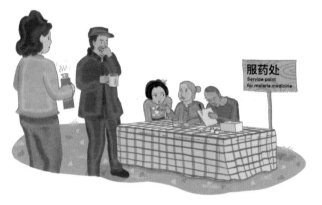

20 世纪 70 年代，传播休止期全民服药
Mass Drug Administration during the non-transmission season for radical cure in the 1970s

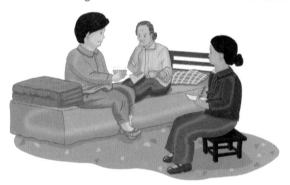

20 世纪 70 年代，走村串户开展服药
Sending Medicine to Villages and Households in the 1970s

图 4-10 大规模人群服药
Figure 4-10 Large-scale Mass Drug Administration

　　大规模人群服药期间，疟疾防治人员经常手提暖壶，身背药箱，走家串户，田间地头，采取"送药到手，看服到口，咽下才走，吐了再补"的服药措施。同时将通俗易懂、朗朗上口的语句，如"疟疾蚊子传，吃药不要钱，得了疟疾病，快找卫生员"等广泛刷写在居民房舍墙上，达到满目皆是的效果，使群众不但抬头可见，一看就懂，过目不忘，而且保留的时间长，效果持久。

　　河南省永城市于 1991 年达到基本消灭疟疾的标准（发病率低于 1 人次 /万），连续 11 年没有本地疟疾病例报告。然而，在 2003 年至 2006 年期间，疟

to gradually achieve the goals of preventing outbreaks, controlling epidemics, reducing incidence, achieving basic elimination, and ultimately eliminating the disease. Large-scale MDA plays a crucial role in this long-term process.

4.9   Let's All Take Medication to Control Malaria

Tips

> When a malaria breaks out, everyone needs to take medicine together to kill all the parasites in their bodies in a short period of time, thus interrupt the disease transmission the disease from spreading to a wider range.

The experience of malaria control programme in China highlights the efficacy of MDA in combating the spread of temperate vivax malaria epidemics in Chinese history, besides treating existing patients. Based on different drug administration purposes, MDA can be divided into preventive MDA and curative MDA. Preventive MDA refers to the intermittent provision of specific anti-malaria drugs or drug combinations during periods of malaria transmission risks and the prevention of malaria occurrence by maintaining therapeutic drug levels in blood. This approach is extensively used in most regions to prevent cases during the transmission season and is applicable to various malaria parasite infections. Curative MDA, by contrast, is typically suitable for *Plasmodium vivax* or *Plasmodium ovale* infections due to existing delayed-type plasmodium parasites in liver. It involves the use of drugs to treat malaria parasites in blood and liver, aiming for complete cure of patients. Generally, curative MDA is given at the beginning or imminent onset of the transmission season to prevent cases from becoming sources of infection. This approach is usually conducted in winter or spring.

To rapidly control the malaria epidemic, province A implemented preventive MDA for over 20 counties affected by the outbreaks. The provincial health department made a plan for MDA, and the fiscal budget allocated funds for drug administration expenses. Province-wide unified procurement and distribution of drugs ensured their availability in various locations. Before the commencement of drug administration, extensive pre-drug administration publicity campaigns were conducted in villages prepared for MDA. Wall posters, banners, and radio broadcasts informed villagers about the timing and target groups of drug administration

疾病例迅速增加；2006 年在 4 个乡镇发现 36 个暴发点；2006 年永城市病例数占全省总病例数的 56.78%。2007 年至 2009 年，对永城市 5 个乡镇 91 个村共 183 688 人进行了大规模人群服药治疗。全程治疗率达 96% 以上。疟疾发病率迅速下降，2011 年报告了最后一例本地疟疾病例，2018 年确认该市消除疟疾。

从实施控制到消除疟疾是一项长期、艰巨的工作任务，需要经过长期、反复防治，逐步达到防止暴发、控制流行、降低发病率、基本消除和最终消除的目标，大规模人群服药治疗在此过程中发挥了重要的作用。

4.9　大家同步服药一起控制疟疾

> **小提示**
>
> 当发生疟疾流行时，需要大家一起来服药，在短时间内把所有人体内的虫子都杀死，这样疾病就流行不起来了。

中国的疟疾防治经验表明，大规模人群服药（mass drug administration，MDA）是中国历史上控制温带型间日疟流行的强有效措施，也是对现症患者治疗的最主要措施。按照服药目的不同，可分为预防性 MDA 和根治性 MDA。预防性 MDA 是指在有疟疾传播风险期间，间歇性地提供某种抗疟药或联合用药，通过保持血液中治疗药物水平来预防疟疾的发生，在大部分地区用于预防病例在传播季节发生，适用于各种疟原虫的感染。根治性 MDA 通常适用于间日疟原虫或卵形疟原虫的感染，使用治疗血液中和肝脏中的疟原虫的药物，以达到完全治愈患者，一般在传播季节开始时或将要到来时对病例进行根治，以防止病例作为传染源进入传播季节，通常在冬季或春季进行。

为快速控制疟疾的流行，A 省对发生疫情的 20 多个县实施预防性人群服药，省卫生厅制定人群服药的方案，财政拨付服药所需的经费，由省级统一

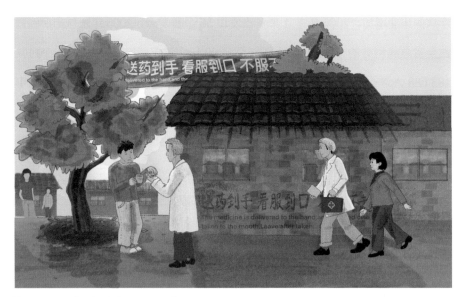

图 4-11 "送药到手，看服到口"
Figure 4-11 "hand the med, watch it fed"

for malaria prevention. A drug delivery team consisting of one doctor from the health center, one village official, and one village doctor visited each household to register the names of individuals requiring drug administration. On the day of the scheduled MDA, the drug delivery team distributed drugs to villagers and supervised their intake. The team adhered to the requirement of "hand the med, watch it fed, won't leave until it's fully swallowed" ensuring compliance throughout the entire treatment course. For those who were temporarily absent or failed to take medicine, the drug delivery team revisited their homes to provide additional doses. Technical guidance and training were provided by provincial, municipal, and county disease prevention and control centers; staff from city, county and township governments also toured villages to monitor drug administration compliance. As a result of the MDA implementation, the incidence rate of malaria significantly decreased compared to the previous year.

购买药品配发至各地。在服药开始前，各个准备开展服药的自然村开展了声势浩大的服药前宣传活动，村子墙上刷制了标语，树上悬挂了横幅，村里的广播站播放着服药要求，使村子里的人们都知道了什么时间需要服预防得疟疾的药以及哪些人需要服药，由1名卫生院医生、1名村干部和1名村医组成的送药小分队逐家逐户地登记需要服药的人员。到了规定统一服药的那天，送药小分队将药品一一送到人们手中，看着他们吃完，按要求做到"送药到手，看服到口，不服不走"，确保了整个治疗过程的服从，对于有些临时外出或没服上药的人，送药小分队还会再次来到他们家中让他们补服药品；省、市、县疾病预防控制中心的技术指导组在各县负责技术培训和指导；市、县和乡政府的工作人员在每个村巡回查看人们的服药情况。随着服药的落实，当年疟疾发病率较上年同期大幅度下降。

5 Treatment

5.1 Recommendations for Timely and Standardized Treatment

Tips

Patients with fever should take a blood test to promptly detect malaria, as early detection is crucial;

Early treatment is more likely to lead to a favorable prognosis, while delayed treatment can be life-threatening.

Medication should be tailored to the patient's condition, with focus on anti-malaria drugs that match the symptoms;

Artemisinin-based injections are the preferred choice for treating critically ill patients.

(1) The key to treating malaria cases is early identification of patients and prompt use of anti-malaria drugs.

(2) The anti-malaria drugs should be administrated according to the severity of the disease. Patients with mild symptoms can be treated with conventional oral drug administrations, while those with severe illness should use artesunate injections or artemether intramuscular injections as early as possible.

(3) Special situations call for special handling. Under specific circumstances, based on typical clinical manifestations and confirmed epidemiological history, artemisinin-based injections in a short period of time (not solely relying on blood test results) after rapid assessment of the patient's condition can significantly reduce the likelihood of developing into severe cases.

5 治 疗

5.1 及时规范治疗的建议

小提示

发热患者要血检，及早发现很关键；

早期治疗易康复，一旦拖延太凶险。

根据病情来用药，抗疟对症抓重点；

青蒿素类注射液，抢救危重是首选。

（1）早期识别患者并能尽快使用抗疟药是治疗疟疾病例的关键。

（2）给药途径按病情轻重来区别对待。症状轻的常规使用口服方剂即可，病情重的，应尽早使用青蒿琥酯注射液静脉推注，或蒿甲醚肌肉注射。

（3）特殊情况特殊处理。在特定的情况下，根据典型的临床表现、明确的流行病学史，快速进行病情评估后，在很短时间内（不单纯依赖血检结果）使用青蒿素类注射液，可大大降低疟疾患者发展成危重症病例可能。

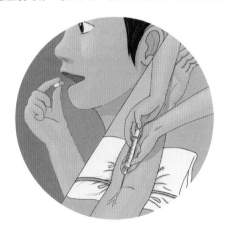

图 5-1 疟疾给药方式

Figure 5-1 Anti-malaria Drugs Administration

Table 5–1   Advantages and Disadvantages of Oral Administration and Intravenous Injection

Route of Medication	Advantages	Disadvantages
Oral Administration	Cost-effective and safe; simple and convenient for patients; patients can self-administer; non-invasive	1. Variable drug absorption efficacy, influenced by gastrointestinal motility, gastric emptying rate, and presence of food in the gastrointestinal tract, etc.; 2. Affected by first-pass metabolism; 3. Unconscious patients cannot adopt oral administration; 4. Inappropriate for patients experiencing vomiting; 5. Slow onset of action; 6. Drugs may be destroyed by digestive enzymes and/or stomach acid; 7. Sublingual administration, which involves administration under the tongue, allows direct absorption into the systemic circulation via blood vessels located beneath the tongue, thereby bypassing first-pass metabolism
Intravenous injection	Immediate effect (suitable for emergent situations); applicable for unconscious patients; bypassing first-pass metabolism; plasma drug concentration is more predictable and accurate compared to other routes	1. Allergic shock may occur; 2. Infection risk; 3. Inconvenient for patients; 4. Pain; 5. Higher cost; 6. Risk of phlebitis or drug leakage; 7. Trained medical personnel for management is required; 8. The drug cannot be stopped once injected; 9. Time-consuming and labor-intensive, such as calculating doses, searching for diluents to be used, checking the compatibility of intravenous drugs, preparing drugs, and administering injections

5.2   Available Anti-Malaria Drugs

Global anti-malaria drugs can be classified into three categories depending upon their functions: anti-malaria drugs to control malaria symptoms, anti-malaria drugs to prevent malaria from recurrence and anti-malaria drugs for prophylactic medication of malaria.

Drugs to control malaria symptoms: dihydroartemisinin, dihydroartemisinin + piperaquine phosphate, artesunate, artesunate + amodiaquine, artesunate

表 5-1　口服用药和静脉注射优缺点

用药途径	优　点	缺　点
口服药	便宜、安全；对患者来说简单而方便；患者可以自行用药；非侵入性	1. 药物吸收效果变化较大，影响药物吸收的因素包括胃肠蠕动、胃排空率以及胃肠道内是否有食物； 2. 受到首关代谢的影响； 3. 无意识的患者不能采用口服途径； 4. 不适用于正在呕吐的患者； 5. 起效缓慢； 6. 药物可能被消化酶和（或）胃酸破坏； 7. 舌下含服途径，用于舌下途径的药物剂型是在舌下给药，药物从位于舌下的血管吸收并直接进入系统循环，从而避免了首关代谢
静脉注射	立即见效（适用于紧急情况）；可以给无意识的患者使用；避免了首关代谢；与其他途径相比，血药浓度可预测和可精确控制	1. 可能出现过敏性休克； 2. 存在感染风险； 3. 对患者不方便； 4. 疼痛； 5. 费用更昂贵； 6. 有静脉炎或药物外渗的风险； 7. 需要训练有素的医护人员来管理； 8. 一旦注射，药物无法停止； 9. 耗费时间和精力，例如需要计算剂量，查找要使用的稀释剂，检查静脉注射药物的相容性，准备药物和注射药物

5.2　现在可用的抗疟药

全球抗疟药物按功用细分，可分为三大类：控制疟疾症状的抗疟药、防止疟疾复发的抗疟药以及预防疟疾的抗疟药。

控制症状药物：双氢青蒿素、双氢青蒿素＋磷酸哌喹，青蒿琥酯、青蒿琥酯＋阿莫地喹、青蒿琥酯＋甲氟喹、蒿甲醚、蒿甲醚＋苯芴醇；奎宁、磷酸氯喹、磷酸哌喹、甲氟喹、阿莫地喹、多西环素、磺胺多辛＋乙胺嘧啶。

防止复发药物：伯氨喹。

预防药物：磷酸氯喹、多西环素、甲氟喹、氯胍、阿莫地喹–磺胺多辛＋乙胺嘧啶、磺胺多辛＋乙胺嘧啶。

+ mefloquine, artemether, artemether + benflumetol; quinine, chloroquine phosphate, piperaquine phosphate, mefloquine, amodiaquine, doxycycline, sulfadoxine + pyrimethamine.

Drugs to prevent malaria recurrence: primaquine.

Drugs for prophylactic medication: chloroquine phosphate, doxycycline, mefloquine, proguanil, amodiaquine-sulfadoxine + pyrimethamine, sulfadoxine + pyrimethamine.

📖 Extended Reading

In 1972, Chinese scientist Tu Youyou and her team successfully extracted artemisinin from *Artemisia annua* leaves, which became the first compound developed in China and has been hailed as milestone in the history of anti-malaria drug research by the international community. Artemisinin anti-malaria drugs only use their derivatives in clinic, including artemether, artesunate and dihydroartemisinin. Such drugs are characterized by fast absorption, extensive distribution and rapid metabolism and excretion, so they need to be administered many times in treatment. Artemisinin is lethal to malaria parasites at all phases of life, and it is the most extensively used drug in clinical treatment of malaria.

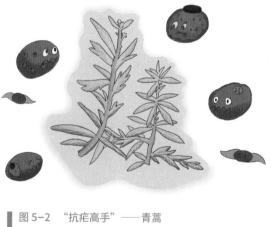

图 5-2 "抗疟高手" ——青蒿
Figure 5-2 "Malarial Killer" – *Artemisia Annua*

5.3 Case 10: A Collection of Traditional Chinese Medicine—The Birth of Artemisinin

Malaria is one of the ancient human diseases, which still threatens human

　　中国科学家屠呦呦团队在 1972 年成功从青蒿叶子中提取分离出具有抗疟活性的青蒿素，成为新中国研制的第一个化学药品，被国际社会誉为抗疟药研究史上的"里程碑"。青蒿素类抗疟药在临床上只用其衍生物，包括蒿甲醚、青蒿琥酯及双氢青蒿素，这类药物具有吸收快、分布广、代谢和排泄迅速的特点，所以治疗时需要多次给药。青蒿素对疟原虫各个生命阶段都是有效的，是目前临床治疗疟疾中应用最为广泛的一种药物。

5.3　案例 10：中医宝典——青蒿素的诞生

　　疟疾是古老的人类疾病之一，至今仍然威胁着人类的健康。在青蒿素问世前，抗疟药以奎宁、氯喹、阿莫地喹等为主。然而，随着药物长期大量使用，疟原虫耐药性的问题逐渐凸显，全球迫切需要新的抗疟药。1967 年，在"523 办公室"的领导下，中国启动了抗疟项目。屠呦呦所在的研究院很快参加到这个项目之中，她被委任为疟疾研究小组组长。第一阶段他们研究了超过 2 000 种中药，发现其中的 640 种可能有抗疟效果。研究员们用小鼠模型评估了从大约 200 种中药里获得的 380 种提取物。然而，过程并没有那么顺利。想要有重大发现谈何容易。一份青蒿提取物给研究工作带来了转机。青蒿提取物很好地抑制了寄生虫的生长。然而，这个发现并没有在之后的实验中重复出来，并且与此前文献中记载的有冲突。为了找到合理的解释，他们翻阅了大量的文献。唯一一篇关于使用青蒿减轻疟疾症状的文献出自葛洪的《肘后备急方》。文中提到："青蒿一握，以水二升渍，绞取汁，尽服之。"

　　这句话给了屠呦呦灵感。为何古人将青蒿"绞取汁"，而不用传统的水煎

health today. Before artemisinin came out, quinine, chloroquine and amodiaquine were the main anti-malaria drugs. However, with the long-term and extensive use of drugs, the problem of malaria parasite resistance gradually emerged, and there was an urgent need for new anti-malaria drugs globally. In 1967, under the leadership of the "523 Office", China launched the anti-malaria project. Tu Youyou's research institute promptly engaged in the project, and she was appointed as the head of the anti-malaria drug research team. In the first phase, they studied over 2,000 traditional Chinese medicines and found that 640 of them might have anti-malaria effects. Researchers used a mouse model to evaluate 380 extracts obtained from approximately 200 traditional Chinese medicines. However, the process was far from smooth. Making significant discoveries was no easy task, until an extract from *Artemisia annua* leaves was found as a turning point in the research. This extract effectively inhibited the growth of the parasite. However, this finding was not replicated in subsequent experiments and conflicted with previous literature. To find a reasonable explanation, they reviewed a vast amount of literature. The only literature on using *Artemisia annua* to alleviate malaria symptoms was from Ge Hong's "The Handbook of Prescriptions for Emergencies". The text mentioned: "Take one grip of *Artemisia annua*, macerated it in two liters of water, wring out the juice and swallow it up."

This sentence inspired Tu Youyou. Why did ancient people extract the juice of *Artemisia annua* instead of using the traditional method of boiling traditional Chinese medicine in water? The answer emerged — they used fresh *Artemisia annua* juice! This enlighten Tu Youyou to realize that the previous ineffective treatments might be due to the conventional "water decoction" method. As high temperatures destroyed the active ingredients in *Artemisia annua*, she adopted a different approach and used low-boiling-point solvents for experiment. This experiment eliminated the acidic part, which had no anti-malaria activity but toxic side effects, and retained the neutral part with strong anti-malaria activity, safety and reliability. This significantly enhanced the efficacy of *Artemisia annua* in preventing and treating malaria while reducing its toxicity to a substantial extent. They then separated the extract into acidic and neutral parts. Finally, in October 1971, they obtained a neutral and non-toxic extract which showed a 100% efficacy against *Plasmodium berghei* infections in mice and *Plasmodium cynomolgi* infected in macaque monkeys. This progress marked a breakthrough in the discovery of artemisinin.

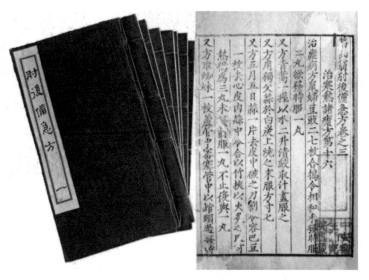

图 5-3　明代（公元 1574 年）葛洪著作《肘后备急方》
Figure 5-3　The Handbook of Prescriptions for Emergencies written by Ge Hong in Ming Dynasty (AD 1574)

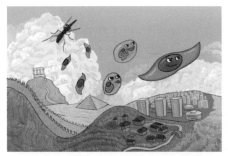
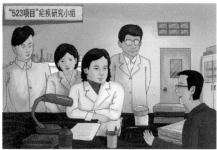
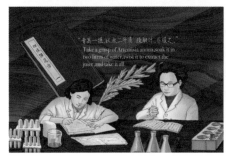
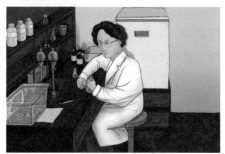

图 5-4　提取青蒿素
Figure 5-4　Extracting Artemisinin

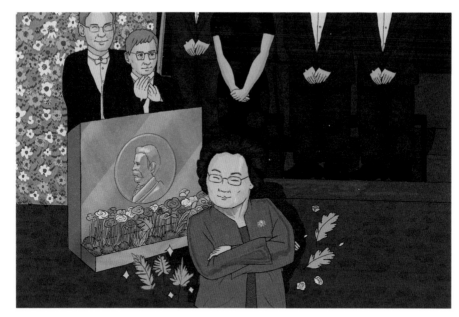

图 5-5　2015 年 12 月，屠呦呦获得诺贝尔奖
Figure 5-5　Tu Youyou won the Nobel Prize in December 2015

Artemisinin, an anti-malaria drug, is derived from *Artemisia annua*, a traditional Chinese medicine. The application of artemisinin and its derivatives, and compound formulations has proposed an effective solution to the global problem of malaria drug resistance. As the preferred treatment for malaria worldwide, artemisinin and its derivatives have relieved the suffering of millions of patients, making a significant contribution to the development of artemisinin. Thus, Tu Youyou, the scientist who led the research on artemisinin, became the first Chinese scientist to win the Nobel Prize in Science for conducting groundbreaking research in China. On October 5, 2015, the Nobel Prize Committee awarded the Nobel Prize in Physiology or Medicine to Tu Youyou and two other scientists.

Chinese medicine is a treasure trove of knowledge, from which artemisinin was discovered. It is a gift from traditional medicine to the world. Researching natural products and developing medicinally valuable substances or modifying them are essential strategies in drug research and new drug development. There are countless treasures in natural products, which require dedicated researchers like Tu Youyou to conduct rigorous research and development, apply them scientifically, and address limitations, for better service to humanity.

熬煮中药之法呢？原来古人用的是青蒿鲜汁！一语惊醒梦中人，屠呦呦意识到以前效果不明显，问题可能出在常用的"水煎"法上。因为高温会破坏青蒿中的有效成分，她随即另辟蹊径采用低沸点溶剂进行实验。这个试验，消除了没有抗疟活性且有毒性副作用的酸性部分，保留了抗疟活性强、安全可靠的中性部分，在明显提高青蒿防治疟疾效果的同时，还大幅降低了它的毒性。随后他们把提取物分离为酸性和中性两部分。终于，在 1971 年 10 月，他们获得了中性无毒的提取物。这份提取物对伯氏疟原虫感染的小鼠和食蟹猴疟原虫感染的猴子有着 100% 的疗效。这个结果标志着青蒿素发现上的突破。

青蒿素是从中国传统药物青蒿中提取的抗疟药物。青蒿素及其衍生物、复方的应用为全球疟疾耐药性难题提供了有效的解决方案。青蒿素及其衍生物作为全球疟疾治疗的首选药物，解除了数百万疟疾患者的病痛，因此在青蒿素研制中作出了突出贡献的屠呦呦成为因为在中国本土进行的科学研究而首次获诺贝尔科学奖的中国科学家。2015 年 10 月 5 日，诺贝尔奖委员会把诺贝尔生理学或医学奖授予屠呦呦等三名科学家。

中国医药学是一个伟大宝库，青蒿素正是从这一宝库中发掘出来的，是传统医学给世界的一份礼物。对天然产物进行研究，针对其开发具有药用价值的物质，或者对天然产物进行改造，是药物研究、新药开发的重要手段。天然药物中有无数瑰宝，这些瑰宝需要像屠呦呦这样的研究者以严谨的态度潜心研究，将其开发出来，以科学的形式为人们所应用，并直面其不足，以致对其进行改造，更好地为人类服务。

📖 Extended Reading

Malaria and the Nobel Prize

(1) Nobel Prize in Physiology or Medicine in 1902: In 1897, Ronald Ross, a British doctor, confirmed that *Anopheles* mosquito was the vector of malaria and expounded the development history of malaria parasites.

(2) Nobel Prize in Physiology or Medicine in 1907: Charles Louis Alphonse Laveran, a French military doctor, discovered malaria parasites in blood cells in 1880.

(3) Nobel Prize in Physiology or Medicine in 1927: Julius Wagner, an Austrian psychiatrist, invented malaria parasites inoculation therapy to treat paralytic dementia caused by syphilis.

(4) Nobel Prize in Chemistry in 1965: Robert Burns Woodward, an American organic chemist, synthesized quinine for the first time and won the Nobel Prize in Chemistry. Quinine became the first-line anti-malaria medicine.

(5) Nobel Prize in Physiology or Medicine in 2015: Tu Youyou, a scientist from China, was awarded the Nobel Prize for her research on artemisinin discovery.

5.4 Recommendations for the Treatment of Severe Malaria Patients

Tips 1

The progression of malaria, particularly *Plasmodium falciparum* malaria, can be extremely sudden. Anyone with a travel history in malaria-endemic regions should seek medical treatment promptly if showing symptoms such as fever, chills, and headache.If confirmed with diagnosis of malaria, standardized anti-malaria drug administration is necessary to prevent the occurrence of severe malaria.

Tips 2

To reduce the mortality rate of cerebral malaria or severe malaria, comprehensive treatment measures must be taken. The treatment of severe malaria should include anti-malaria therapy, supportive treatment, symptomatic management, complications treatment, as well as intensive care, prevention of secondary infections, and other measures.

1. Carry out malaria surveillance among mobile populations

This is the key to detecting malaria cases. Conduct detailed inquiry into the

📖 拓展阅读

疟疾与诺贝尔奖

（1）1902 年诺贝尔生理学或医学奖：英国医生罗纳德·罗斯（Ronald Ross）于 1897 年证实按蚊是疟疾的传播媒介，阐明疟原虫的发育史。

（2）1907 年诺贝尔生理学或医学奖：法国军医夏尔·路易·阿方斯·拉韦朗（Charles Louis Alphonse Laveran）于 1880 年发现血细胞中的疟原虫。

（3）1927 年诺贝尔生理学或医学奖：奥地利精神科医生尤利乌斯·瓦格纳（Julius Wagner）发明了疟原虫接种疗法来治疗梅毒导致的麻痹性痴呆。

（4）1965 年诺贝尔化学奖：美国的有机化学家罗伯特·伯恩斯·伍德沃德（Robert Burns Woodward），因首次人工合成了奎宁而获得诺贝尔化学奖，奎宁一度成为抗疟一线用药。

（5）2015 年诺贝尔生理学或医学奖：中国科学家屠呦呦凭借对青蒿素的研究成果获得了诺贝尔奖。

5.4 疟疾重症患者的治疗建议

小提示 1

疟疾，特别是恶性疟的病情进展可能会非常突然，有疟疾流行地区旅居史的，一旦出现发热、寒战、头痛等症状时务必及时就医。如果确诊疟疾要规范服用抗疟药，这样才能防止重症疟疾的发生。

小提示 2

要降低脑型疟或重症疟疾的病死率，必须采取综合性的治疗措施。重症疟疾的治疗应包括抗疟治疗、支持治疗、对症处理、并发症治疗以及加强护理、防止合并感染等措施。

1. 开展流动人口疟疾监测

这是发现疟疾病例的关键所在。加强患者流行病史的询问，特别是对来

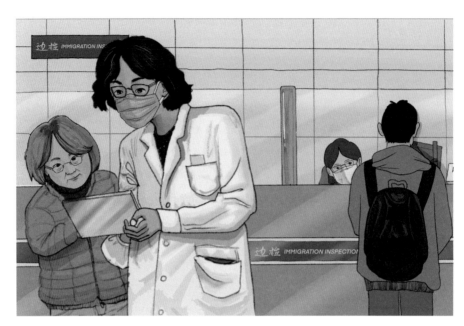

图 5-6　海关入境疟疾监测
Figure 5-6　Surveillance of Imported Malaria in Customs

epidemiological history of personnel, especially among the high-risk populations of migrant workers, students, residents, and travelers from malaria-endemic regions, timely blood sampling for malaria parasite detection is crucial for early detection, early diagnosis, and early treatment to prevent the disease from progressing from mild to severe cases.

2. Cerebral malaria is the primary killer of severe malaria

The clinical manifestations of severe malaria mainly include coma, confusion, severe anemia, acute renal insufficiency, pulmonary edema or acute respiratory distress syndrome, hypoglycemia, circulatory failure or shock, metabolic acidosis, etc. These symptoms can be observed in cerebral malaria. Cerebral malaria is mostly developed from *plasmodium falciparum* malaria, influencing mostly young children and patients with no immunity, with a poor prognosis.

3. Timely and correctly use anti-malaria drugs

In the treatment of severe malaria cases, especially cerebral malaria, highly effective and rapid-acting anti-malaria medicines should be given by intravenous or intramuscular routes. The WHO gives priority to the use of artesunate injection as the preferred drugs for the treatment of all severe malaria cases. In the absence

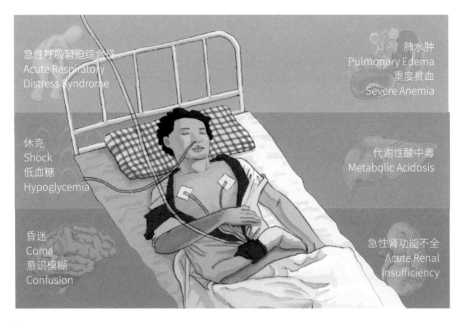

急性呼吸窘迫综合征
Acute Respiratory
Distress Syndrome

休克
Shock
低血糖
Hypoglycemia

昏迷
Coma
意识模糊
Confusion

肺水肿
Pulmonary Edema
重度贫血
Severe Anemia

代谢性酸中毒
Metabolic Acidosis

急性肾功能不全
Acute Renal
Insufficiency

图 5-7　脑型疟临床表现
Figure 5-7　Clinical Manifestations of Cerebral Malaria

自疟疾流行区域的务工、学习、居住、旅行的重点人群，要及时采血检查疟原虫，做到早发现、早诊断、早治疗，避免病情从轻症发展成重症。

2. 脑型疟是重症疟疾的主要致死原因

重症疟疾的临床表现主要有昏迷、意识模糊、重度贫血、急性肾功能不全、肺水肿或急性呼吸窘迫综合征、低血糖、循环衰竭或休克、代谢性酸中毒等，以上症状均可见于脑型疟；脑型疟绝大部分由恶性疟发展而成，以幼童及无免疫力的患者为多见，预后凶险。

3. 及时、正确使用抗疟药物

治疗重症疟疾病例，特别是脑型疟时，必须采用杀虫作用高效、快速的抗疟药，进行静脉注射或肌肉注射给药。世界卫生组织优先推荐使用青蒿琥酯注射剂作为治疗所有重症疟疾的首选药物，在没有青蒿琥酯注射剂的情况

of artesunate injection, artemether or quinine injection can also be used to save patients. The largest randomized clinical trial conducted to date on severe *Plasmodium falciparum* malaria cases has shown that compared with quinine injection, intravenous or intramuscular injection of artesunate can significantly reduce mortality. Meanwhile, artemisinin is simpler and safer to use.

(1) Artesunate injection: Artemether, a derivative of artemisinin, appears as a white crystalline powder, which is dissolved in sodium bicarbonate (5%) to form sodium artesunate, and then diluted with approximately 5ml of 5% glucose solution. It is injected intravascular or intramuscular into the anterior thigh.

The treatment regimen consists of intravenous injection of 2.4mg/kg of artesunate, followed by another dose at 0, 12, and 24 hours. If the patient wakes up and can eat after treatment, an Artemisinin based combination therapy （ACTs） course of oral administration is adopted for 3 days.

(2) Artemether injection: The activity of artemether is 2-3 times more than that of its main metabolite, dihydroartemisinin. Artemether can be administered as an oil-based intramuscular injection or orally. In severe *Plasmodium falciparum* malaria, the concentration of the parent compound dominates after intramuscular injection, while exogenous artemisinin is rapidly and almost totally hydrolyzed into dihydroartemisinin. After intramuscular injection, the absorption of artemether may be slower and less stable than that of water-soluble artesunate, while water-soluble artesunate is rapidly and reliably absorbed after intramuscular injection. These pharmacological advantages may help explain the clinical superiority of artesunate in the treatment of severe malaria. Artemether is dissolved in oil (peanut, sesame) and injected intramuscularly into the anterior thigh.

Treatment dosage: The initial dose of artemether is 3.2mg/kg bw[①] (anterior thigh). The maintenance dose is 1.6mg/kg bw daily.

(3) Supportive treatment: Appropriate fluid administration, adequate glucose supplementation, and correction of metabolic acidosis and water-electrolyte balance are required. Patients with erythrocytes < 2.5 million/μL receive blood transfusions. The use of adrenal cortex hormones (10-20mg of dexamethasone or 100-300mg of hydrocortisone) on the 1st day is effective in controlling high fever and promoting recovery, but daily use is not necessary.

(4) Symptomatic management and prevention and cure of complications: promptly controlling high fever and seizures, promoting consciousness, and

---

① bw: body weight.

下也可采用蒿甲醚注射剂或奎宁注射剂抢救患者。迄今对重症恶性疟疾进行的最大随机临床试验表明，与注射奎宁相比，静脉或肌肉注射青蒿琥酯可显著降低死亡率，同时，青蒿素使用起来更简单和安全。

（1）青蒿琥脂注射液。青蒿琥酯是一种青蒿素的衍生物，白色结晶性粉末，溶解在碳酸氢钠（5%）中形成青蒿琥酯钠，然后用大约 5ml 5% 的葡萄糖稀释溶液，在大腿前部进行静脉注射或肌肉注射。

治疗方案为：青蒿琥酯注射液 2.4mg/kg 静脉推注，0 小时、12 小时和 24 小时各 1 次，若患者苏醒并能进食，则改以青蒿素为基础的联合疗法（ACTs）1 个疗程 3 天口服。

（2）蒿甲醚注射液。蒿甲醚的活性是其主要代谢物双氢青蒿素的 2～3 倍。蒿甲醚可作为油基肌肉注射或口服。在严重恶性疟中，肌内注射后母体化合物的浓度占主导地位，而肠外青蒿素能迅速且几乎完全水解成双氢青蒿素。肌肉注射后，蒿甲醚的吸收可能比水溶性青蒿琥酯更慢、更不稳定，而水溶性青蒿琥酯在肌肉注射后吸收迅速、可靠。这些药理优势可能解释了青蒿琥酯治疗重症疟疾的临床优势。将蒿甲醚溶解于油（花生、芝麻）中，通过肌肉注射入大腿前部。

治疗剂量：蒿甲醚的初始剂量为 3.2mg/kg bw[1] 肌注（大腿前）。维持剂量为每日肌注 1.6mg/kg bw。

（3）支持治疗：要适量输液，补充足量的葡萄糖，纠正代谢性酸中毒和维持水电解质平衡。红细胞 ＜ 250 万 /μL 者给予输血。第 1 天使用肾上腺皮质激素（地塞米松 10～20mg 或氢化可的松 100～300mg），对控制高热、促进病情恢复效果颇佳，但不必每天使用。

（4）对症处理和并发症防治：尽快控制高热和抽搐，促进患者清醒，这

———————
[1] bw：体重。

achieving these goals are essential for preventing complications. Early detection and timely management of complications are key to raising the cure rate.

Common severe complications include brain damage, gastrointestinal damage, shock, hemolysis, severe liver/kidney damage, pulmonary edema, severe anemia, abnormal bleeding, hypoglycemia, acidosis, etc.

Management of complications: paying attention to timely fever and sedation control; managing brain edema; managing central respiratory failure, maintaining respiratory tract unimpeded, and oxygen inhalation; avoiding heart failure, reducing cardiac load, and preventing pulmonary edema; avoiding shock, adjusting blood volume appropriately; correcting acidosis and heart failure; managing metabolic acidosis promptly; avoiding hemolysis, using adrenal cortex hormones appropriately, adequate fluid infusion, and diuresis; managing renal failure; and blood transfusion for severe anemia.

📖 Extended Reading

【Case】Mr. Wen, a 43-year-old male, departed for Cameroon in Africa to explore business opportunities in April of 2014 and returned to China on December 25, 2015. He had a history of malaria while working abroad. On December 27, he visited the outpatient department of neurology in the local county people's hospital due to "dizziness, neck and shoulder pain, and insomnia." As the patient did not have a fever at the time and did not provide the attending doctor with a history of working abroad in Africa, the doctor did not consider malaria. Instead, a cranial and cervical CT scan was performed, and the initial diagnosis was cervical spondylosis due to three-joint vertebral disc herniations seen on the cervical CT. The patient was prescribed medications such as Xuesaitong Capsules to treat and observe at home.

The patient was found lying in bed at home by his family at 6 pm on December 30, unresponsive, incontinent of bowel and bladder. They immediately called 120 and the patient was sent to the local county people's hospital for treatment. Based on the information provided that the patient had a history of working in Africa, the patient was diagnosed with *Plasmodium falciparum* malaria upon admission. The diagnosis was severe cerebral malaria, and the patient was given intravenous injection of artesunate, together with symptomatic treatment such as oxygen therapy and volume expansion. On December 31, the patient's condition worsened, with tachypnea, weakness, and deepening coma. While continuing the anti-malaria treatment with artesunate injection, the patient was given a tracheal intubation and mechanical ventilation when respiratory distress persisted. During the symptomatic management, albumin was used to maintain osmotic pressure of blood colloid, hormones were administered to alleviate cerebral edema, antibiotics were given for infection control, and erythrocyte transfusion was performed to correct anemia. After the above treatment,

是预防并发症的基本措施。及早发现、及时处理并发症，是提高治愈率的关键。

常见的严重并发症有脑损害、胃肠损害、休克、溶血、严重的肝/肾损害、肺水肿、严重贫血、异常出血、低血糖、酸中毒等。

并发症的处理：注意及时退热镇静；处理脑水肿；处理中枢性呼吸衰竭，保持呼吸道畅通，氧气吸入；注意避免出现心力衰竭，减轻心脏负荷，防止肺水肿；避免出现休克，适时补充血容量；注意纠正酸中毒和心功能不全；注意及时处理代谢性酸中毒；注意避免出现溶血，适时使用肾上腺皮质激素，充足输液和利尿；注意处理肾功能衰竭；重度贫血时应予以输血。

📖 拓展阅读

【案例】温某某，男，43岁，2014年4月出发到非洲喀麦隆淘金，于2015年12月25日回国，境外务工期间有疟疾病史。12月27日因"头晕、颈部及肩背部酸痛、失眠"到当地县人民医院神经内科门诊就诊，因当时患者未有发热症状，患者亦未给接诊医生提供外出非洲务工史，因此接诊医生未往疟疾方面考虑，给予行颅脑和颈椎CT检查，因颈椎CT见三节椎间盘膨出，初步诊断颈椎病，开血塞通胶囊等相关药物回家治疗观察。

患者12月30日18时被其家属发现躺于自家床上，呼之不应，大小便失禁，即呼叫120送至当地县人民医院救治。根据家属提供的"患者有外出非洲淘金史"信息，入院后急查血涂片检出恶性疟，诊断为重症脑型疟，即给予青蒿琥脂注射液静脉注射处理，同时给予吸氧、扩容等对症治疗。12月31日患者病情加重，呼吸急促、乏力，昏迷加深，在继续用青蒿琥脂注射液抗疟治疗的同时，予气管插管术，呼吸无改善后即予呼吸机辅助通气。期间采取应用白蛋白维持血液胶体渗透压平衡，用激素辅助减轻脑水肿，予抗生素抗感染治疗，予输红细胞纠正贫血等对症处理。经上述治疗后患者病情逐渐好转，2016年1月12日患者可自行进食，精神佳，血涂片检查未找到疟原虫，复查血常规、肝肾功能、心肌酶、胸片等情况良好，达到临床治愈予以办理出院。

the patient's condition gradually improved. By January 12, 2016, the patient was able to feed himself, exhibited good spirits, and a blood smear examination did not show malaria parasites. Repeated blood tests, liver and kidney function tests, myocardial enzyme tests, and chest X-rays showed normal results. The patient was clinically cured and discharged from the hospital.

5.5   How to Use Drugs to Cure Malaria?

Tips 1

The principle of standard drug administration is timely, reasonable, safe and sufficient.

Tips 2

It is crucial to diagnose malaria early and undergo comprehensive treatment for effective results; rational and standard drug use, combined with joint treatment, is essential; individualized dosage adjustments should be made according to the patient's body weight to guarantee scientifically sound therapeutic regimens.

Four major principles should be followed in the treatment and oral administration of malaria cases:

1. Early diagnosis and rapid and effective treatment

Plasmodium falciparum malaria can rapidly develop into a life-threatening disease, particularly in populations with no immunity or low immunity. Severe *Plasmodium falciparum* malaria can easily progress to cerebral malaria and cause death if not treated in a prompt manner. Therefore, all plans should guarantee early diagnosis and rapid, effective treatment within 24-48 hours after the appearance of malaria symptoms.

2. Rational use of anti-malaria drugs

To minimize the emergence of drug resistance, curtail the unnecessary use of anti-malaria drugs, and better identify other febrile diseases in the context of changing malaria epidemiology, it is crucial to guarantee that anti-malaria drugs are used only for patients genuinely suffering from malaria, while promoting the consistent completion of a full course of treatment.

5.5 怎样用药才能治好疟疾？

┌─── **小提示 1** ─────────────────────────────
│
│ 规范服药的原则即及时、合理、安全、足量。
│
└──

┌─── **小提示 2** ─────────────────────────────
│
│ 疟疾发现要尽早，全程治疗效果好；用药合理又规范，联合治疗不单干；患
│ 者体重有差别，剂量方案讲科学。
│
└──

在疟疾病例的治疗和服药过程中，要遵循以下四大原则。

1. 早期诊断和迅速有效的治疗

恶性疟可迅速发展为危及生命的疾病，特别是在没有免疫力或免疫力低下的人群中，严重恶性疟如果不及时治疗，很容易发展为脑型疟并引起患者死亡。因此，各项方案应确保在疟疾症状出现后 24 ～ 48 小时内获得早期诊断和迅速、有效的治疗。

2. 合理使用抗疟药物

为了减少耐药性的出现，限制抗疟药物的不必要使用，并在疟疾流行病学发生变化的背景下更好地识别其他发热性疾病，确保抗疟药物只对真正患有疟疾的患者使用，同时提倡坚持一个完整的疗程，这是非常重要的。

3. 联合治疗

预防或延迟耐药性的产生对于国家和全球控制和最终消除疟疾战略的成功至关重要。为保护当前和未来的抗疟药物，都应使用至少两种具有不同作用机制的有效抗疟药物（联合疗法）进行治疗。

4. 根据体重科学给药

为了延长抗疟药的治疗效果并确保所有患者都有平等的治愈机会，必须

3. Combined therapy

The prevention or containing drug resistance development is essential for the success of national and global malaria control and eradication strategies. To safeguard current and future anti-malaria drugs, treatment should be used at least two effective anti-malaria drugs with different mechanisms of action (combination therapy).

4. Scientific Administration by Weight

To prolong the efficacy of anti-malaria drugs and guarantee equal cure opportunities for all patients, it is essential to guarantee the quality of anti-malaria drugs and provide them at optimal doses. Treatments should aim to maximize the likelihood of cure and minimize the transmission of post-treatment infections. To achieve this goal, dose regimens should be based on patient weight and provide effective anti-malaria drug concentrations over a sufficient duration.

The drugs used for treating malaria cases are specifically as below.

1. Recommended medicines for treatment of *Plasmodium falciparum* malaria

(1) Artemether + benflumetol tablets

(2) Artesunate + amodiaquine tablets

(3) Artesunate + mefloquine tablets

(4) Dihydroartemisinin + piperaquine phosphate tablets

(5) Artesunate + sulfadoxine-pyrimethamine tablets

2. Recommended medicines for treatment of non-severe *Plasmodium vivax* malaria and *Plasmodium ovale* malaria

(1)14-day therapy with chloroquine phosphate and primaquine

(2) 8-day therapy with chloroquine phosphate and primaquine

(3) 8-day therapy with piperaquine phosphate and primaquine

(4) 8-day therapy with artemisinin compound and primaquine

3. Recommended use for treatment of *Plasmodium malariae* malaria

(1) 3-day therapy with chloroquine phosphate

(2) 3-day therapy with piperaquine phosphate

(3) 3-day therapy with artemisinin compound

4. Recommended medicines for treatment of mixed infection

Artemisinin-based combination therapy is effective for all malaria parasites, as is the choice of treatment for mixed infection. The therapeutic regimen is artemisinin-based combination therapies (ACTs) + primaquine.

确保抗疟药物的质量，并给患者提供最佳剂量。治疗应最大限度地提高治愈的可能性，并最大限度地减少治疗后感染的传播。为实现这一目标，剂量方案应基于患者的体重，并在足够的时间内提供有效的抗疟药物浓度。

疟疾病例的治疗所使用的药物如下。

1. 恶性疟的治疗推荐使用

（1）蒿甲醚＋苯芴醇片

（2）青蒿琥酯＋阿莫地喹片

（3）青蒿琥酯＋甲氟喹片

（4）双氢青蒿素＋磷酸哌喹片

（5）青蒿琥酯＋磺胺多辛－乙胺嘧啶片

2. 非重症间日疟、卵形疟治疗推荐使用

（1）磷酸氯喹、伯氨喹 14 日疗法

（2）磷酸氯喹、伯氨喹 8 日疗法

（3）磷酸哌喹、伯氨喹 8 日疗法

（4）青蒿素类复方加伯氨喹 8 日疗法

3. 三日疟治疗推荐使用

（1）磷酸氯喹 3 日疗法

（2）磷酸哌喹 3 日疗法

（3）青蒿素类复方 3 日疗法

4. 混合感染的治疗推荐使用

以青蒿素为基础的联合疗法对所有疟原虫都有效，对混合感染的治疗选择也是如此，治疗方案为以青蒿素为基础的联合疗法（ACTs）＋伯氨喹。

📖 Extended Reading

Detailed Regimen for Use of anti-malaria Drugs

1. Recommended use for treatment of *Plasmodium falciparum* malaria

(1) Artemether + benflumetol tablet: the total dose of artemether is 5-24 mg/kg body weight(bw), and the total dose of benflumetol is 29-144 mg/kg bw. The recommended administration regimen is artemether + benflumetol, twice a day for 3 days (6 times in total). Ideally, the interval between the first two doses should be 8 hours. Pregnant women, lactating women and those who are allergic to any ingredients in the compound prescription are forbidden to take this drug. This drug cannot be used to treat severe malaria or prevent malaria.

(2) Artesunate + amodiaquine tablet: a combination tablet with a fixed dose, which contains 25 + 67.5mg, 50 + 135mg or 100 + 270mg of artesunate and amodiaquine respectively.

Daily dose of 4 (2-10) mg/kg bw artesunate + 10 (7.5-15) mg/kg bw amodiaquine, once a day, for 3 consecutive days. It is suitable for the rescue of cerebral malaria and all types of severe malaria cases, with good tolerance and no significant adverse reactions.

(3) Artesunate + mefloquine tablet: a formulation with a fixed dose, including children's tablets containing 25mg of artesunate and 55mg of mefloquine hydrochloride (equivalent to 50mg of mefloquine base) and adult tablets containing 100mg of artesunate and 220mg of mefloquine hydrochloride (equivalent to 200mg of mefloquine base).

Daily dose of 4 (2-10) mg/kg bw artemisinin + 8.3 (5-11) mg/kg bw mefloquine, once a day, for 3 consecutive days. It is suitable for the rescue of cerebral malaria and all types of severe malaria cases.

(4) Dihydroartemisinin + piperaquine phosphate tablet: the currently available fixed-dose combination tablets contain 40mg of dihydroartemisinin + 320mg of piperaquine phosphate, as well as children's tablets containing 20mg of dihydroartemisinin + 160mg of piperaquine phosphate.

For adults and children with a body weight ≥ 25kg, the target dose (range) every day is 4 (2-10)mg/kg bw dihydroartemisinin and 18 (16-27) mg/kg bw piperaquine phosphate, once a day, for 3 consecutive days. For children with a body weight less than 25kg, the target dose and range every day are 4 (2.5-10) mg/kg bw dihydroartemisinin and 24 (20-32) mg/kg bw piperaquine phosphate, once a day, for 3 consecutive days.It is used to treat *Plasmodium falciparum* malaria and *Plasmodium vivax* malaria, with a relatively strong killing effect on *Plasmodium* asexual body, rapidly killing malaria parasites and thus controlling symptoms. There are few adverse reactions, chiefly caused by piperaquine phosphate.

(5) Artesunate + sulfadoxine/pyrimethamine tablet: Currently available ones are bubble-packaged scratch tablets, containing 50mg of artesunate and fixed-dose combination tablets containing 500mg of sulfadoxine + 25mg of pyrimethamine. There is no fixed-dose combination.

抗疟药使用详细方案

1. 恶性疟的治疗推荐使用

（1）蒿甲醚＋苯芴醇片：蒿甲醚总剂量为 5 ～ 24mg/kg bw，苯芴醇总剂量为 29 ～ 144mg/kg bw。推荐给药方案：蒿甲醚＋苯芴醇，每日 2 次，共 3 天（共 6 次）。理想情况下，前 2 次剂量应该间隔 8 小时。孕妇、哺乳期妇女、对复方中任何成分过敏者禁用。该药不用于治疗严重疟疾或预防疟疾。

（2）青蒿琥酯＋阿莫地喹片：一种固定剂量的组合片剂，分别含有 25+67.5mg、50+135mg 或 100+270m 青蒿琥酯和阿莫地喹。

每天 4（2 ～ 10）mg/kg bw 青蒿琥酯 +10（7.5 ～ 15）mg/kg bw 阿莫地喹，每天 1 次，连续 3 天。适用于脑型疟疾及各种危重疟疾的抢救，耐受性好，无明显副反应。

（3）青蒿琥酯＋甲氟喹片：一种固定剂量的配方，包括含有 25mg 青蒿琥酯和 55mg 甲氟喹盐酸盐（相当于 50mg 甲氟喹碱）的儿童片剂和含有 100mg 青蒿琥酯和 220mg 甲氟喹盐酸盐（相当于 200mg 甲氟喹碱）的成人片剂。

每天 4（2 ～ 10）mg/kg bw 青蒿素 +8.3（5 ～ 11）mg/kg bw 甲氟喹，每天 1 次，连续 3 天。适用于脑型疟及各种危重疟疾的抢救。

（4）双氢青蒿素＋磷酸哌喹片：目前提供的固定剂量组合片剂含有 40mg 双氢青蒿素 +320mg 磷酸哌喹，以及含有 20mg 双氢青蒿素 +160mg 磷酸哌喹的儿童片剂。

体重为 25kg 及以上的成人和儿童，目标剂量（范围）为每天 4（2 ～ 10）mg/kg bw 双氢青蒿素和每天 18（16 ～ 27）mg/kg bw 磷酸哌喹，每天 1 次，连续 3 天。体重轻于 25kg 的儿童的目标剂量和范围是每天 4（2.5 ～ 10）mg/kg bw 双氢青蒿素和每天 24（20 ～ 32）mg/kg bw 磷酸哌喹，每天 1 次，连续 3 天。用于治疗恶性疟和间日疟，对疟原虫无性体有较强的杀灭作用，能迅速杀灭疟原虫，从而控制症状。不良反应较少，主要由磷酸哌喹引起。

（5）青蒿琥酯＋磺胺多辛 / 乙胺嘧啶片：目前有水泡包装的划痕片，含 50mg 青蒿琥酯和固定剂量组合片，含 500mg 磺胺多辛 +25mg 乙胺嘧啶。没有固定剂量的组合。

Daily dose of 4 (2-10) mg/kg bw artesunate, once a day, for 3 consecutive days, and a single dose of sulfadoxine/pyrimethamine on the 1st day of at least 25/1.25 (25-70/11.25-3.5) mg/kg bw.Effective against *Plasmodium falciparum* malaria and *Plasmodium vivax* erythrocytes in the early stage, it can also inhibit the development of malaria parasites in mosquitoes, thus blocking transmission. It is commonly used in clinical practice for preventing malaria and treating recurrence during the non-transmission season.

2. Treatment of non-severe *Plasmodium vivax* malaria and *Plasmodium ovale* malaria

To treat *Plasmodium* vivax and *Plasmodium* ovale malaria, both the World Health Organization (WHO) and China recommend a combination of chloroquine and primaquine. The goal of this treatment is to eliminate the *Plasmodium* parasites within red blood cells and to clear liver-stage hypnozoites, thereby preventing relapse. However, the WHO recommends a 14-day therapy, while China follows an 8-day therapy. The main differences between the two therapies lie in the duration of treatment and the dosage of primaquine. Specifically, the dosage of chloroquine used in China is the same as the WHO's recommendation, but China's daily dose of primaquine (22.5 mg/day) is higher than the WHO's recommended dose (15 mg/day). Additionally, China's 8-day primaquine therapy is shorter than the WHO's 14-day therapy, and both of them can achieve a good eradication effect. 8-day regimen seems to be more effective in improving patient adherence and compliance because of the shorter duration of the therapy.

(1) 14-day therapy of chloroquine phosphate and primaquine. The total oral dose of chloroquine for adults is 1 200 mg (base, the same below): 600 mg on the 1st day taken at a draught or in two times, 300 mg each time; 300 mg taken at a draught on the 2nd and 3rd days. The total oral dose of primaquine for adults is 210 mg: 15 mg every day, taken at a draught, from the 1st day of taking chloroquine phosphate, for 14 consecutive days.

(2) 8-day therapy of chloroquine phosphate and primaquine. The total oral dose of chloroquine for adults is 1 200 mg (base, the same below): 600 mg on the 1st day taken at a draught or in two times, 300 mg each time; 300 mg taken at a draught on the 2nd and 3rd days. The total oral dose of primaquine for adults is 180 mg: 22.5 mg every day, taken at a draught, from the 1st day of taking chloroquine phosphate, for 8 consecutive days.

In the susceptible regions of chloroquine, adults and children suffering *Plasmodium vivax* malaria, *Plasmodium ovale* malaria, *Plasmodium malariae* malaria or *Plasmodium knowlesi* malaria without complications should be treated with ACT or chloroquine phosphate. In the drug-resistant regions of chloroquine phosphate, adults and children suffering *Plasmodium vivax* malaria, *Plasmodium ovale* malaria, *Plasmodium malariae* malaria or *Plasmodium knowlesi* malaria without complications (except pregnant women in the first trimester) should be treated with ACT.

每日 4（2～10）mg/kg bw 青蒿琥酯，每天 1 次，连续 3 天，并且在第 1 天磺胺多辛／乙胺嘧啶单次给药至少 25/1.25（25～70/11.25～3.5）mg/kg bw。对恶性疟及间日疟原虫红细胞前期有效，也能抑制疟原虫在蚊体内的发育，故可阻断传播，临床上常用于预防疟疾和休止期抗复发治疗。

2. 非重症间日疟、卵形疟的治疗

治疗间日疟和卵形疟，世界卫生组织（WHO）和中国均推荐氯喹和伯喹联合用药，其目的是杀灭红细胞内的疟原虫及清除肝内的休眠体，防止出现复发。但是，世界卫生组织推荐 14 日疗法，而中国采用 8 日疗法，两者的主要区别在于疗程的长短和伯氨喹使用剂量的不同，其中中国的氯喹用量与 WHO 推荐的相同，但中国的伯氨喹每日用量（22.5 mg）较 WHO 推荐的剂量（15mg）要大；而伯氨喹疗程中国推荐 8 日疗法，较 WHO 推荐的 14 日疗法要短，都能达到很好的根治效果。8 日疗法因缩短了疗程，似乎更能提高感染者全程服药率和依从性。

（1）磷酸氯喹、伯氨喹 14 日疗法。氯喹成人口服总剂量 1 200mg（基质，下同），第 1 日 600mg 顿服或分 2 次服，每次 300mg，第 2、3 日各顿服 300mg。伯氨喹成人总剂量 210mg，从服用磷酸氯喹的第 1 日起，每天顿服 15 mg，连服 14 日。

（2）磷酸氯喹、伯氨喹 8 日疗法。氯喹成人口服总剂量 1 200mg（基质，下同），第 1 日 600mg 顿服或分 2 次服，每次 300mg，第 2、3 日各顿服 300mg。伯氨喹成人总剂量 180 mg，从服用磷酸氯喹的第 1 日起，每天顿服 22.5 mg，连服 8 日。

在氯喹易感地区，用 ACT 或磷酸氯喹治疗无并发症的间日疟、卵形疟、三日疟或诺氏疟成人和儿童。在磷酸氯喹耐药地区，用 ACT 治疗无并发症的间日疟、卵形疟、三日疟或诺氏疟成人和儿童（妊娠早期的孕妇除外）。

（3）磷酸哌喹、伯氨喹 8 日疗法。哌喹成人口服总剂量 1 200mg（基质，下同），第 1 日 600mg 顿服或分 2 次服，每次 300mg；第 2、3 日各顿服 300mg。伯氨喹成人口服总剂量 180mg，从服用磷酸哌喹的第 1 日起，每日顿服 22.5mg，连服 8 日。

在 G6PD 缺乏的人群中，考虑通过给予伯氨喹基础剂量 0.75mg/kg bw，每周一次，持续 8 周来预防复发，同时密切医疗监督潜在的伯氨喹引起的不良血液反应。

(3) 8-day therapy of piperaquine phosphate and primaquine. The total oral dose of piperaquine for adults is 1200mg (matrix, the same below): 600mg on the 1st day taken at a draught or at two times, 300mg each time; 300mg taken at a draught on the 2nd and 3rd days. The total dose of primaquine taken orally is 180mg: 22.5mg every day, taken at a draught, from the 1st day of taking piperaquine phosphate, for 8 consecutive days.

In the population with G6PD deficiency, it is considered to prevent recurrence by giving a basic dose of 0.75mg/kg bw primaquine once a week for 8 consecutive weeks, and to closely monitor the potential adverse blood reactions caused by primaquine.

(4) 8-day therapy with artemisinin compound and primaquine

1) Dihydroartemisinin piperaquine phosphate tablets. The total dose of dihydroartemisinin piperaquine phosphate tablets is 8 tablets, each containing 40mg of dihydroartemisinin and 171.4mg of piperaquine phosphate (matrix). It is taken orally for 2 days, with 2 tablets for the 1st dose, and 2 tablets taken at 8 hours, 24 hours and 32 hours respectively.

2) Artesunate amodiaquine tablets. The total dose of artesunate amodiaquine tablets is 6 tablets, each containing 100mg of artesunate and 270mg of amodiaquine (matrix), 1 time per day, 2 tablets per time, for 3 consecutive days.

3) Artemisinin piperaquine tablets. The total dose of artemisinin piperaquine tablets is 4 tablets, each containing 62.5mg of artemisinin and 375mg of piperaquine phosphate (matrix), once a day, 2 tablets/ time, for 2 consecutive days.

3. Recommended use for treatment of *Plasmodium malariae* malaria

(1) 3-day therapy with chloroquine phosphate

The total dose of chloroquine phosphate (chloroquine matrix) is 1200mg (8 tablets, each containing 150mg of chloroquine phosphate matrix), taken orally for 3 days: 600mg (4 tablets) on the 1st day, taken at a draught or at two times, with 300mg (2 tablets) each time; once on the 2nd and 3rd day respectively, 300mg (2 tablets) each time.

(2) 3-day therapy with piperaquine phosphate

The total dose of piperaquine phosphate (piperaquine matrix) is 1200mg (8 tablets, each containing 150mg of piperaquine phosphate matrix), which is taken orally for 3 days, 600mg (4 tablets) on the 1st day, taken at a draught or at two times, or 300mg (2 tablets) each time; once on the 2nd and 3rd day respectively, 300mg (2 tablets) each time.

(3) Therapy with artemisinin compound

1) Dihydroartemisinin piperaquine phosphate tablets. The total dose of dihydroartemisinin piperaquine phosphate tablets is 8 tablets, each containing 40mg of dihydroartemisinin and 171.4mg of piperaquine phosphate (matrix). It is taken orally for 2 days, with 2 tablets for the 1st dose, and 2 tablets taken at 8 hours, 24 hours and 32 hours respectively.

（4）青蒿素类复方加伯氨喹8日疗法

1）双氢青蒿素磷酸哌喹片。双氢青蒿素磷酸哌喹片总剂量8片，每片含双氢青蒿素40mg、磷酸哌喹（基质）171.4mg。分2日口服，首剂口服2片，8小时、24小时、32小时后各口服2片。

2）青蒿琥酯阿莫地喹片。青蒿琥酯阿莫地喹片总剂量6片，每片含青蒿琥脂100mg、阿莫地喹（基质）270mg。每日1次，2片/次，连服3日。

3）青蒿素哌喹片。青蒿素哌喹片总剂量4片，每片含青蒿素62.5mg、磷酸哌喹（基质）375mg。每日1次，每次2片，连服2日。

3. 三日疟治疗推荐使用

（1）磷酸氯喹3日疗法

磷酸氯喹（氯喹基质）总剂量1200 mg（8片，每片含磷酸氯喹基质150mg），分3日口服，第1日600mg（4片）顿服，或分2次口服，每次300mg（2片）；第2日和第3日各服1次，每次300mg（2片）。

（2）磷酸哌喹3日疗法

磷酸哌喹（哌喹基质）总剂量1200 mg（8片，每片含磷酸哌喹基质150mg），分3日口服，第1日600mg（4片）顿服，或分2次口服，每次300mg（2片）；第2日和第3日各服1次，每次300mg（2片）。

（3）青蒿素类复方疗法

1）双氢青蒿素磷酸哌喹片。双氢青蒿素磷酸哌喹片总剂量8片，每片含双氢青蒿素40mg、磷酸哌喹（基质）171.4mg。分2日口服，首剂口服2片，8小时、24小时、32小时后各口服2片。

2）青蒿琥酯阿莫地喹片。青蒿琥酯阿莫地喹片总剂量6片，每片含青蒿琥脂100mg、阿莫地喹（基质）270mg。每日1次，2片/次，连服3日。

3）青蒿素哌喹片。青蒿素哌喹片总剂量4片，每片含青蒿素62.5mg、哌喹（基质）375mg。每日1次，每次2片，连服2日。

2) Artesunate amodiaquine tablets. The total dose of artesunate amodiaquine tablets is 6 tablets, each containing 100mg of artesunate and 270mg of amodiaquine (matrix), once a day, 2 tablets per time, for 3 consecutive days.

3) Artemisinin piperaquine tablets. The total dose of artemisinin piperaquine tablets is 4 tablets, each containing 62.5mg of artemisinin and 375mg of piperaquine (matrix), once a day, 2 tablets/time, for 2 consecutive days.

5.6　Case 11　What to Do if Feeling Unwell after Taking Medicines ?

Tips 1

The side effects are mild, and it is mainly intended to promote metabolism, and if there is no relief, go to the hospital for diagnosis and treatment in time.

Tips 2

If you experience nausea, vomiting, abdominal pain, diarrhea, dizziness, headache, drowsiness, blurred vision, migraine, tinnitus, rash, dermatitis, or itching after taking anti-malaria drugs, it may be due to adverse reactions to the drugs.

Typically, the side effects of taking the therapeutic dose are mild and can disappear spontaneously after stopping the medication. Therefore, if you experience uncomfortable symptoms after taking anti-malaria drugs, it is recommended to drink plenty of boiled water to promote drug metabolism in your body, pause medication, and observe for a period of time to see if symptoms gradually disappear. If it is not suitable to stop medication, you can take medicine after meals to reduce stomach irritation and alleviate abdominal discomfort. You may also consult a doctor to adjust the route of administration, such as switching from oral to intravenous administration, or replacing it with similar drugs with milder adverse reactions. If the above measures are ineffective or symptoms become more severe, it is essential to seek prompt medical diagnosis and treatment.

Case 11

On May 30, 2013, Mr. Li, a 28-year-old male, was diagnosed with *Plasmodium*

5.6 案例 11 服药后不舒服怎么办？

小提示 1

不良反应轻微以促进代谢方法为主，没有缓解及时到医院诊治。

小提示 2

如果服用抗疟药后有恶心、呕吐、腹痛、腹泻、头昏、头痛、嗜睡、视力模糊、头痛、耳鸣、皮疹、皮炎、皮肤瘙痒等情况，可能是出现了用药后的不良反应。

通常服用治疗量的副反应较轻，停药后可自行消失，因此，服用抗疟药出现不舒服的症状后，建议大量喝开水，促进药物在体内的代谢，同时暂停服药，观察一段时间，看症状是否慢慢好转；如不宜停药，服药可改为在饭后服，减少口服药物对胃的刺激，减轻胃部不适感；也可在医生指导下调整用药途径，例如由口服改为静脉注射等，或是换为其他副反应较轻的同类药物。如果以上措施都没有效果，或是症状越来越严重，需要尽快到医院进行诊治。

案例 11

李某某，男，28 岁，2013 年 5 月 30 日在 S 县疾控中心被诊断为恶性疟，给予口服青蒿琥酯 + 阿莫地喹抗疟治疗，"布洛芬"退热，用药第二天起患者腹胀腹痛明显，伴随多次呕吐，到 S 县人民医院就诊后，医生建议抗疟药饭后服用并加用护胃药物，患者遵医嘱，但腹胀、腹痛、呕吐症状未缓解；6 月 1 日患者再来就诊时医生考虑口服用药副反应过大，同时体温仍不退，继续口服药效果不佳，亦容易导致病情恶化，于是调整为住院给予静脉用青蒿琥酯，患者病情迅速得到控制，6 月 3 日治愈出院。

蓝某某，男，44 岁，2014 年 6 月 19 日被诊断为间日疟，G6PD 正常，

falciparum malaria at the CDC of County S. He was given oral artesunate and amodiaquine for anti-malaria treatment along with ibuprofen for fever reduction. From the 2nd day of medication, he experienced abdominal distension and pain, accompanied by multiple vomits. After visiting the S County People's Hospital, the doctor recommended taking anti-malaria drugs after meals and adding stomach protection drugs. However, his symptoms of abdominal distension, pain, and vomiting did not improve. On June 1, considering that the oral administration causes severe adverse reactions and the patient's body temperature still remained high, and continuous oral medication was ineffective and could easily lead to worsening conditions, the doctor switched the treatment to intravenous artesunate. The patient's condition was quickly controlled, and he was discharged on June 3 after cured.

Mr. Lan, a 44-year-old male, was diagnosed with *Plasmodium vivax* malaria on June 19, 2014, with normal G6PD. He was prescribed chloroquine/primaquine tablets for radical treatment. However, the patient began to have symptoms such as dizziness, fatigue, abdominal distension, nausea, and vomiting the second day after taking the medication. He went to the County People's Hospital for consultation, complaining that he felt worse after taking the medication than before, and requested to stop or change the medication. At that time, the only available radical treatment for *Plasmodium vivax* malaria in the county was chloroquine/primaquine tablets, and the patient's adverse reactions were relatively mild, mainly psychological issues. The doctor explained the importance of anti-malaria drugs and suggested taking them after meals, separating the administration of chloroquine and primaquine in appropriate time intervals, and visiting the doctor promptly if symptoms worsened. The patient accepted the advice and was able to complete the medication without any difficulty. His symptoms were relieved, with no recurrence since then.

Summary: From 2013 to the end of 2021, the County People's Hospital treated more than 2,140 malaria cases, with 1,739 cases admitted. The majority of these cases were treated with injectable artesunate, while oral medication cases were fewer. In the early stages (in 2013), the most common and widespread adverse reaction to oral artesunate amodiaquine tablets was gastrointestinal discomfort, which was relatively severe, leading to patient resistance and low compliance. In response, County S adjusted its treatment approach to intravenous injection of artesunate. From 2015 onwards, dihydroartemisinin piperaquine tablets were used, with reduced adverse reactions, and most malaria cases were tolerable. The number of cases taking oral anti-malaria tablets significantly increased.

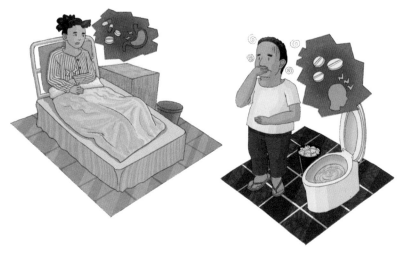

图 5-8　服药不良反应
Figure 5-8　Adverse Reactions after Taking the Drugs

给予氯喹 / 伯氨喹片根治，但患者用药后第二天就开始出现头昏、乏力、腹胀、恶心、呕吐等症状，患者到 S 县人民医院咨询，诉用药后比没用药之前还难受，要求停药或换药，根据当时县里只有氯喹 / 伯氨喹片根治间日疟药物，而且患者口服用药后出现的副反应相对较轻，主要是心理上的问题，遂跟患者说明用抗疟药的重要性，同时建议饭后服用，氯喹和伯氨喹适当分开，在不同时间段服用，如果症状加重及时就诊，患者接受建议并能顺利服完上药，症状缓解，此后未见复发。

小结： S 县人民医院从 2013 年至 2021 年底，共治疗疟疾患者 2 140 多人次，其中共 1 739 人次住院，绝大部分都是使用注射用青蒿琥酯，口服用药的病历较少，早期（2013 年时）时使用青蒿琥酯阿莫地喹片口服时副反应最常见比较普遍的是胃肠道反应，且较为严重，所以用此口服用药时患者抗拒较多，导致依从性较差，根据此情况，S 县在救治过程中调整为静脉输用青蒿琥酯注射液。2015 年后改为使用双氢青蒿素哌喹片，副反应减少，疟疾病例都能忍受，口服抗疟药片剂例数明显增多。

5.7   Various Interventions to Prevent Recurrence

Apart from prophylactic medication for emergency population to eliminate the sources of infection, Province implemented a population wide radical cure campaign in the spring of the following year to consolidate the prevention and control efforts, strengthened case detection and disposed of transmission sites simultaneously. Clinical doctors and laboratory doctors in malaria-endemic regions receive malaria diagnosis and treatment annually. Upon detecting a malaria case, they immediately initiated the following tasks:

(1) Case treatment: Providing immediate medication or treatment free of charge.

(2) Case reporting: The doctors report the case information at the online surveillance system for disease prevention and infectious diseases in China within 24 hours. This system is operated in township health centers, as well as in various county-level, city-level, and province-level hospitals. Cases detected by the village clinical doctors will be immediately reported to the township health center by phone.

(3) Case investigation: Staff from the county-level CDC_s will verify the case information within 3 days. They will conduct an epidemiological investigation on the patient and his/her residence to determine the sources of infection and transmission risk. Besides, patients will be advised to avoid being bitten by mosquitoes during medication to prevent from infecting others.

(4) Disposal of transmission sites: Within 7 days, staff from the county-level disease prevention and control institution will carry out health education for timely medical treatment against mosquitoes and fever, mosquito killing by insecticides, prophylactic medication and other disposal measures of endemic sites in the residence of cases and surrounding regions in consideration of the local settings. Through these measures, patients are no longer infected, so that the transmission is cut off.

5.8   Case 12   Important Health Management Approach — Health Education

Come together to spread awareness against malaria

April 25 is the World Malaria Day. In 2021, the global mortality of malaria was up to 619,000, and Africa continued to bear over 90% of the global burden of malaria

5.7　多种措施预防再发

除了应急性开展人群预防性服药清除传染源外，为巩固防治效果，A省在疟疾流行的次年春季再次实施根治性人群服药。同时加强病例的发现和疫点处置。疟疾流行区的医疗机构临床医生和检验医生每年都接受疟疾诊治的培训，他们每发现一例疟疾病例，就立即启动下列工作。

（1）病例治疗：立即给予免费的药物治疗。

（2）病例报告：医生于当天（24小时内）将病例的信息通过网络上报到中国疾病预防传染病监测系统，这个系统在每个乡的卫生院以及各个县级、市级和省级的医院都有。如果是村卫生室的医生发现病例，会立即电话上报乡级卫生院。

（3）病例调查：县级疾病预防控制机构的工作人员在看到病例的信息后，会在3天内对病例开展核实和流行病学调查，从而判断患者的感染来源和传播风险，同时告知患者在服药期间避免被蚊子叮咬，以防传染给别人。

（4）疫点处置：县级疾病预防控制机构的工作人员在7天内对病例居住地及周围一定区域根据实际情况开展人群防蚊灭蚊和发热及时就医的健康教育、杀虫剂灭蚊、预防性服药等疫点处置措施。通过上述措施，使患者不再传染蚊子、没有蚊子被传染，也没有被感染的蚊子传染其他人，从而实现没有人被传染，切断疫情的传播。

5.8　案例12　重要的健康管理模式——健康教育

共筑疟疾防范意识

每年4月25日是世界防治疟疾日，2021年全球疟疾死亡总人数达61.9万，非洲继续承受全球90%以上的疟疾疾病负担。尽管迄今已采取了许多干预措施，但由于社会、经济、政治、文化、战乱等诸方面的阻力，仍无法有效遏

diseases. Despite numerous interventions, it remains challenging to effectively curb the malaria transmission in Nigeria, Democratic Republic of Congo, Niger, Tanzania,and other countries owing to the resistance of societal, economic, political and cultural factors, and civil conflict. Another overlooked factor is that these interventions lay more emphasis on reducing severe malaria and mortality through improved medical treatment, neglecting the interaction between human health and the surrounding environment. Malaria health education, especially in remote regions with limited medical conditions, can raise people's awareness of malaria prevention, driving behavioral changes from an individual level to a family level, and eventually radiating to the societal level, thus reducing the burden of malaria diseases. Therefore, it is crucial to conduct health education and protect individuals from being infected with malaria parasites. The take home messages for malaria are as below.

(1) Malaria is a parasitic disease caused by infection with malaria parasites, which is preventable and curable. The typical symptoms of malaria include chills, fever, and sweating. Severe malaria patients may also experience coma, delirium, and neck stiffness, which can be life-threatening.

(2) There are four types of malaria parasites on human body, namely *Plasmodium vivax, Plasmodium malariae, Plasmodium falciparum* and *Plasmodium ovale*.

(3) The transmission vector for malaria is *Anopheles* mosquitoes, which begin their blood-sucking activities 0.5 to 2 hours after sunset and can last until 5 a.m. on the next day. The peak blood-sucking period usually occurs in the first half of the night. *Anopheles Gambiae* and *Anopheles arabiensis* mosquitoes are the main malaria vectors in sub-Saharan Africa.

(4) Human beings are generally susceptible to all sorts of human malaria parasites. Newborns in high malaria-endemic regions can acquire antibodies from their mothers through the placenta, but these antibodies disappear after three months, making them easily susceptible. The highest incidence rate occurs within the first two years, after which natural infections result in enhanced immunity, thus reducing the severity of the disease and the frequency of infections. Generally, residents over 25 years old in high malaria-endemic regions have a certain degree of immunity to malaria.

(5) The best way to prevent malaria is to prevent mosquito bites and prohibit malaria patients from donating blood.

(6) In malaria-endemic regions, long-lasting insecticide-treated insecticide-

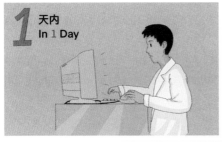
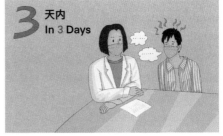
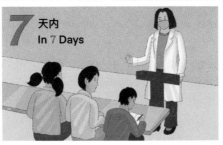

图 5-9 疟疾病例报告与疫点处置的"1-3-7"工作规范
Figure 5-9 Malaria Case Management and the "1-3-7" approach

制尼日利亚、刚果金、尼日尔、坦桑尼亚等国家的疟疾疫情。而另一个被忽视的原因，是干预措施更多地侧重于通过提升医疗救治来降低重症疟疾，减少死亡率，而忽视了健康水平的提升是人与周边环境相互作用的结果。疟疾健康教育，尤其是对于医疗条件落后的偏远地区，有助于提高人们对疟疾的防范意识，进而从意识层面驱动行为的改变，再从个人影响到家庭，乃至向社会层面辐射，从而降低疟疾的负担。因此，做好健康教育、保护个人不被感染上疟原虫极为重要。健康教育的核心知识点如下。

（1）疟疾是一种感染疟原虫引起的，可防可治的寄生虫病，发病的典型症状是发冷、发热和出汗。重症疟疾患者还可见昏迷、谵语、脖硬，危及生命。

（2）寄生于人体的疟原虫主要有四种，即间日疟原虫、三日疟原虫、恶性疟原虫和卵形疟原虫。

（3）疟疾的传播媒介是按蚊，吸血活动始于日落后 0.5～2 小时，可持续至黎明 5 点，吸血高峰通常在上半夜。冈比亚按蚊和阿拉伯按蚊是非洲撒哈

treated nets used at night can prevent mosquito bites and kill mosquitoes simultaneously.

(7) Using safe doses of insecticides not only affect the nets but act on indoor environments where mosquitoes rest, e.g., walls, ceilings, and windows, lowering the rate of mosquito bites to a large extent.

(8) Individuals who have recently traveled to malaria-endemic regions or have a history of living or traveling in malaria-endemic regions and experience high fever, headache, muscle ache, abdominal discomfort, and chills should seek medical attention promptly for diagnosis and treatment.

(9) When visiting a doctor, patients should actively inform the attending doctor about their living and traveling history in malaria-endemic regions.

(10) If diagnosed with malaria, it is crucial to complete the full course of treatment as prescribed by the doctor and take medicine in full doses, to avoid the recurrence or drug resistance.

(11) Those who spend the night in high malaria-endemic regions during the endemic season must take medicine for prophylaxis.

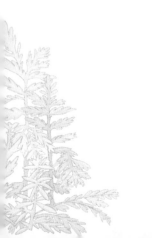

拉以南地区的主要疟疾传播媒介。

（4）人体对各种人类疟原虫普遍易感，高疟区初生儿可经胎盘自母体获得抗体，3 个月后抗体消失而易感，两岁以内的儿童发病率最高，此后由于自然感染后免疫力增强，故感染轻，发病少；一般高疟区 25 岁以上的居民，对疟疾有一定的免疫力。

（5）预防疟疾最好的办法是防止蚊子叮咬和禁止疟疾患者献血。

（6）在疟疾流行区，夜间使用杀虫剂处理的长效蚊帐能在防止蚊虫叮咬的同时杀灭蚊虫。

（7）使用安全剂量的杀虫剂不仅能作用于蚊帐，还能通过室内滞留喷洒，作用于墙面、天花板、窗户等户内蚊虫停栖的地方，能在很大程度上降低蚊虫叮咬率。

（8）近期去过疟疾流行区或有疟疾流行区旅居史的个人，一旦出现高烧、头痛、肌肉酸痛、胃部不适及寒战时，须及时就医，尽快诊断及治疗。

（9）就诊时应主动告诉接诊医生自己有疟疾流行区旅居史。

（10）确诊疟疾后，应按照医嘱全程、足量服药，避免出现复发或耐药。

（11）流行季节在高疟区过夜必须服药预防。

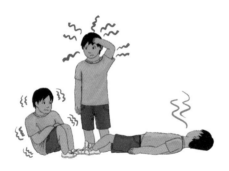

感染疟疾的典型症状为发冷、发热和出汗
Typical symptoms of malaria infection include chills, fever and sweating

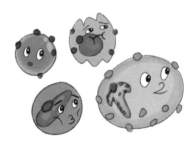

四种寄生于人体的疟原虫
Four types of malaria parasites on human body

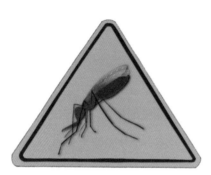

按蚊是疟疾传播媒介
Anopheles mosquitoes are vectors of malaria

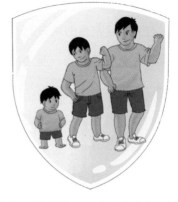

高疟区初生儿和中青年有一定疟疾免疫力
Newborns and young people in high malaria-endemic regions have certain malaria immunity

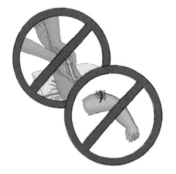

防止蚊子叮咬，禁止疟疾患者献血
Prevent mosquito bites and prohibit malaria patients from donating blood

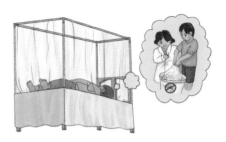

夜间使用长效蚊帐
Use long-lasting insecticide-treated nets at night

图 5-10　疟疾健康教育知识要点
Figure 5-10　Key Points of Malaria-Related Health Education Knowledge

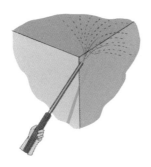

室内滞留喷洒，降低蚊虫叮咬率
Indoor residual spraying lowers the rate
of mosquito bites

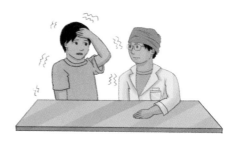

有疟疾流行区旅居史时，
出现发热、头痛、寒战等不适，及时就医
Promptly seek medical attention when
feeling unwell such as fever, headache and
chills, after having a history of living and
traveling in malaria-endemic regions

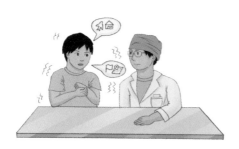

主动告知医生疟疾流行区旅居史
Inform the doctor of the traveling history to
malaria-endemic regions

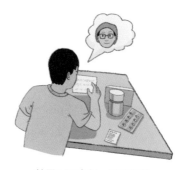

按照医嘱全程、足量服药
Take medicine throughout the whole
course and in full dose according to the
prescription

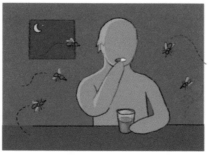

流行季节在高疟区过夜可以服药预防疟疾
Take medicine to prevent when staying
overnight in high endemic regions during
transmission season

References

[1] Chow CY. Malaria vector in China ［J］. Chin J Entomol，1991，Special Publ
(6)：67-79.

[2] Disease Prevention and Control Bureau of the Ministry of Health. Handbook of
Malaria Prevention and Control [M]. Beijing: People's Medical Publishing House,
2007:1-295.

[3] Tang Linhua, Gao Qi. Malaria Control and Eradication in China [M]. Shanghai:
Shanghai Scientific & Technical Publishers, 2013:1-197.

[4] Writing Group of National Medical Center for Infectious Diseases, Li Lanjuan,
Zhang Wenhong, et al. Guidelines for Malaria Diagnosis and Treatment ［J］.
Chinese Journal of Parasitology and Parasitic Diseases, 2022,40(04): 1-9.

[5] Gong Zhenyu, Gong Xunliang. Overview of Global Prevention and Control of
Malaria in 2015 [J]. Disease Surveillance, 2016, 31(02):174-176.

[6] Choi L, Majambere S, Wilson AL. Larviciding to prevent malaria transmission[J].
Cochrane Database Syst Rev, 2019, 8(8):CD012736.

[7] Kellen WR, Meyers CM. Bacillus sphaericus Neide as a pathogen of mosquitoes[J].
J Invertebr Pathol, 1965, 7(4): 442-448.

[8] Regis L, da Silva SB, Melo-Santos MA. The use of bacterial larvicides in mosquito
and black fly control programmes in Brazil[J]. Mem Inst Oswaldo Cruz. 2000;95
Suppl 1:207-210.

[9] Berker N. Microbial control of mosquitoes:management of the upper Rhine
mosquito population as a model programme[J]. Parasitology Today,1997, 13
(12)：485-487.

[10] Wang Rongrong, Tang Linhua. Research Progress on the Role of Bacillus
Sphaericus in Prevention and Control of Vector Mosquitoes [J]. Parasitic
Diseases Foreign Medical Sciences, 2005, 32(2):76-79.

参考文献

[1] Chow CY. Malaria vector in China［J］. Chin J Entomol，1991，Special Publ (6):67-79.

[2] 卫生部疾病预防控制局 . 疟疾防治手册 [M]. 北京：人民卫生出版社，2007:1-295.

[3] 汤林华，高琪 . 中国疟疾的控制与消除 [M]. 上海：上海科学技术出版社，2013:1-197.

[4] 国家传染病医学中心撰写组，李兰娟，张文宏，等 . 疟疾诊疗指南 [J]. 中国寄生虫学与寄生虫病杂志 , 2022, 40(04):1-9.

[5] 龚震宇，龚训良 . 2015 年全球疟疾防控概况 [J]. 疾病监测，2016, 31(02):174-176.

[6] Choi L, Majambere S, Wilson AL. Larviciding to prevent malaria transmission[J]. Cochrane Database Syst Rev, 2019, 8(8):CD012736.

[7] Kellen WR, Meyers CM. Bacillus sphaericus Neide as a pathogen of mosquitoes[J]. J Invertebr Pathol, 1965, 7(4): 442-448.

[8] Regis L, da Silva SB, Melo-Santos MA. The use of bacterial larvicides in mosquito and black fly control programmes in Brazil[J]. Mem Inst Oswaldo Cruz. 2000; 95 Suppl 1:207-210.

[9] Berker N．Microbial control of mosquitoes：management of the upper Rhine mosquito population as a model programme[J]．Parasitology Today, 1997, 13(12): 485-487．

[10] 王蓉蓉，汤林华 . 球形芽孢杆菌在媒介蚊虫防制中作用的研究进展 [J]. 国外医学（寄生虫病分册），2005, 32(2):76-79.

[11] Fillinger U, Lindsay SW. Suppression of exposure to malaria vectors by an order of magnitude using microbial larvicides in rural Kenya [J]. Trop Med Int Health. 2006, 11(11):1629-1642.

[12] Zhou Guangchao, Huang Fang, Zhou Shuisen, et al. Malaria Situation and Evaluation on Different Malaria Prevention and Control Measures in Yongcheng City [J]. Journal of Pathogen Biology, 2009, 4(6):449-452.

[13] Zhang Liang, Ma Xiaoyan. The Formation and Enlightenment of the Concept of "Patriotic Public Health Campaign" in the Early Days of the Founding of New China - An Investigation Centered on People's Daily [J]. Historical Research in Anhui, 2021, (05):160-168.

[14] Li Zidian. Overview of Research on Patriotic Public Health Campaign in Recent Years [J]. Beijing Party History, 2010, No.182(03):25-30.

[15] Shi Mingli, Wu Zhishao, Xu Lifan. Thoughts on the Sustainable Development Strategy of Patriotic Public Health Campaign in Rural Regions in the New Era [J]. Chinese Primary Health Care, 2007, No.254(03):27-29.

[16] Yang Liqun. Barefoot Doctors: the Back of An Era [D]. Shanxi University, 2015.

[17] Long Chang'an, Wang Xuewei. On the State Building of the Barefoot Doctor [J]. Journal of Xinzhou Teachers University, 2018, 34(04):50-55.

[18] Zhu Wenwei. On the Phenomenon of "Barefoot Doctors" and the Rural Health System Reform in China [J]. Intelligence, 2014(14):303-305.

[19] Li Haihong Mao Zedong's Theory and Practice of Barefoot Doctors [J]. Journal of Northwest University (Natural Science Edition), 2013, 43(03):504-509.

[20] Zhang D, Unschuld PU. China's barefoot doctor: past, present, and future[J]. Lancet. 2008 Nov 29;372(9653):1865-1867. doi: 10.1016/S0140-6736(08)61355-0. Epub 2008 Oct 17. PMID: 18930539.

[21] Xu S, Hu D. Barefoot Doctors and the "Health Care Revolution" in Rural China: A Study Centered on Shandong Province[J]. Endeavour. 2017 Sep;41(3):136-145. doi: 10.1016/j.endeavour.2017.06.004. Epub 2017 Jul 8. PMID: 28693889.

[22] Rosenthal MM, Greiner JR. The Barefoot Doctors of China: from political creation to professionalization[J]. Hum Organ. 1982 Winter;41(4):330-41. doi: 10.17730/humo.41.4.h01v12784j114357. PMID: 10299059.

[11] Fillinger U, Lindsay SW. Suppression of exposure to malaria vectors by an order of magnitude using microbial larvicides in rural Kenya [J]. Trop Med Int Health. 2006, 11(11):1629-1642.

[12] 周广超，黄芳，周水森，等 . 永城市疟疾疫情分析及防治效果评价 [J]. 中国病原生物学杂志，2009, 4(6):449-452.

[13] 张亮，马晓艳 . 新中国成立初期"爱国卫生运动"概念的形成及启示——以《人民日报》为中心的考察 [J]. 安徽史学，2021, (05):160-168.

[14] 李自典 . 近年来关于爱国卫生运动研究综述 [J]. 北京党史，2010, No.182 (03):25-30.

[15] 史明丽，吴智韶，许立凡 . 新时期农村爱国卫生运动可持续发展策略的思考 [J]. 中国初级卫生保健，2007, No.254(03):27-29.

[16] 杨立群 . 赤脚医生：一个时代的背影 [D]. 山西大学，2015.

[17] 龙长安，汪雪微 . 国家建设视野中的赤脚医生探讨 [J]. 忻州师范学院学报，2018, 34(04):50-55.

[18] 朱文伟 . 论"赤脚医生"现象与中国农村卫生体制改革 [J]. 才智，2014(14): 303-305.

[19] 李海红 . 毛泽东之赤脚医生的理论与实践探究 [J]. 西北大学学报 (自然科学版)，2013, 43(03):504-509.

[20] Zhang D, Unschuld PU. China's barefoot doctor: past, present, and future[J]. Lancet. 2008 Nov 29;372(9653):1865-1867. doi: 10.1016/S0140-6736(08)61355-0. Epub 2008 Oct 17. PMID: 18930539.

[21] Xu S, Hu D. Barefoot Doctors and the "Health Care Revolution" in Rural China: A Study Centered on Shandong Province[J]. Endeavour. 2017 Sep;41(3):136-145. doi: 10.1016/j.endeavour.2017.06.004. Epub 2017 Jul 8. PMID: 28693889.

[22] Rosenthal MM, Greiner JR. The Barefoot Doctors of China: from

[23] Koplan JP, Hinman AR, Parker RL, et al. The barefoot doctor: Shanghai County revisited[J]. Am J Public Health. 1985 Jul;75(7):768-70. doi: 10.2105/ajph.75.7.768. PMID: 4003652; PMCID: PMC1646317.

[24] Wen C. Barefoot doctors in China[J]. Nurs. Dig. 1975 Jan-Feb;3(1):26-8. PMID: 12259447.

[25] Li LA. The edge of expertise: Representing barefoot doctors in Cultural Revolution China[J]. Endeavour. 2015 Sep-Dec;39(3-4):160-7. doi: 10.1016/j.endeavour.2015.05.007. PMID: 27064158.

[26] Shi L. Health care in China: a rural-urban comparison after the socioeconomic reforms[J]. Bull World Health Organ. 1993;71(6):723-36. PMID: 8313490; PMCID: PMC2393531.

[27] Wang D, Chaki P, Mlacha Y, et al. Application of community-based and integrated strategy to reduce malaria disease burden in southern Tanzania: the study protocol of China-UK-Tanzania pilot project on malaria prevention and control[J]. Infect Dis Poverty. 2019 Jan 8;8(1):4. doi: 10.1186/s40249-018-0507-3. PMID: 30646954; PMCID: PMC6334450.

[28] Expert Advisory Committee on Malaria, Ministry of Health. Great Achievements Have Been made in Prevention and Control of Malaria in Jiangsu, Shandong, Henan, Anhui and Hubei Provinces in the Past 20 years [J]. Journal of Pathogen Biology, 1993: 1.

[29] Shang Leyuan. Report on Joint Prevention and Control of Malaria in Jiangsu, Shandong, Henan, Anhui and Hubei Provinces [J]. Journal of Disease Control & Prevention, 1998(02): 92-93.

[30] Wu Xingrong. Analysis on the Role and Significance of the 20th anniversary of Joint Prevention and Control of Malaria in Five Provinces [J]. Chinese Journal of Parasitology and Parasitic Diseases, 1995, 13(S1): 115-118.

[31] Qian Huilin, Tang Linhua. Achievements and Prospects of Prevention and Control against Malaria in China in the Past 50 Years [J]. Chinese Journal of Epidemiology, 2000, 21(3): 225-227.

[32] Kong Xiangli, Liu Ying, Wang Weiming, et al. Retrospective Analysis of the Effectiveness of Joint Prevention and Control of Falciparum Malaria in Jiangsu,

political creation to professionalization[J]. Hum Organ. 1982 Winter;41(4):330-41. doi: 10.17730/humo.41.4.h01v12784j114357. PMID: 10299059.

[23] Koplan JP, Hinman AR, Parker RL, et al. The barefoot doctor: Shanghai County revisited[J]. Am J Public Health. 1985 Jul;75(7):768-70. doi: 10.2105/ajph.75.7.768. PMID: 4003652; PMCID: PMC1646317.

[24] Wen C. Barefoot doctors in China[J]. Nurs. Dig. 1975 Jan-Feb;3(1):26-8. PMID: 12259447.

[25] Li LA. The edge of expertise: Representing barefoot doctors in Cultural Revolution China[J]. Endeavour. 2015 Sep-Dec;39(3-4):160-7. doi: 10.1016/j.endeavour.2015.05.007. PMID: 27064158.

[26] Shi L. Health care in China: a rural-urban comparison after the socioeconomic reforms[J]. Bull World Health Organ. 1993;71(6):723-36. PMID: 8313490; PMCID: PMC2393531.

[27] Wang D, Chaki P, Mlacha Y, et al. Application of community-based and integrated strategy to reduce malaria disease burden in southern Tanzania: the study protocol of China-UK-Tanzania pilot project on malaria control[J]. Infect Dis Poverty. 2019 Jan 8;8(1):4. doi: 10.1186/s40249-018-0507-3. PMID: 30646954; PMCID: PMC6334450.

[28] 卫生部疟疾专家咨询委员会 . 苏、鲁、豫、皖、鄂五省廿年来疟防工作取得巨大成绩 [J]. 中国寄生虫病防治杂志，1993(6): 1-3.

[29] 尚乐园 . 苏鲁豫皖鄂五省疟疾联防情况汇报 [J]. 疾病控制杂志，1998(02)：92-93.

[30] 吴兴荣 .5 省疟疾联防 20 周年的作用与意义浅析 [J]. 中国寄生虫学与寄生虫病杂志，1995, 13(S1): 115-118.

[31] 钱会霖，汤林华 . 中国五十年疟疾防治工作的成就与展望 [J]. 中华流行病

Anhui and Henan Provinces [J]. China Tropical Medicine, 2016, 16(10): 986-988.

[33] Shang Leyuan, Gao Qi, Liu Xin, et al. Evaluation on the Effect of Cooperative Malaria Control in Five Provinces of Central China in 30 Years [J]. Journal of Pathogen Biology, 2006(01): 51-53.

学杂志，2000, 21(3): 225-227.

[32] 孔祥礼，刘颖，王伟明，等 . 苏皖豫三省恶性疟联防成效回顾性分析 [J].
中国热带医学，2016, 16(10): 986-988.

[33] 尚乐园，高棋，刘新，等 . 苏、鲁、豫、皖、鄂五省疟疾联防 30 年效果
评价 [J]. 中国病原生物学杂志，2006(01): 51-53.

Afterword

The idea for this popular science book was first conceived on September 27, 2021. At that time, China had just received certification from the World Health Organization for the elimination of malaria. There was a call for discussion on how to share China's experience in malaria elimination with our African counterparts and how to jointly build a Community of Health for Mankind. Against this backdrop, five experts from different organizations, including the Shanghai Association for Science and Technology, Shanghai Scientific and Technical Publishers, and the National Institute of Parasitic Diseases of the Chinese Center for Disease Control and Prevention (Chinese Center for Tropical Diseases Research), had a brainstorming meeting at the Shanghai Science Hall, who reached a consensus: the five organizations would collaborate to develop a book that could serve as both a textbook for malaria health education in Africa, and to share China's experience in malaria elimination with African professionals of malaria control.

We established a simple yet profound goal to use bilingual popular science to disseminate China's valuable experience in malaria control and elimination, accumulated over many years, to more countries and regions. This would help people around the world better understand and respond to this long-standing threat to human health. To achieve this, we formed a diverse team comprising malaria experts, writers, young illustrators, and editors. After multiple virtual and in-person discussions, we decided to adopt a bilingual format in both Chinese and English, accompanied by rich illustrations, to show readers how Chinese citizens and experts actively participate in malaria control, how health facilities effectively respond to malaria outbreaks, and how local governments coordinate and manage malaria control efforts, among other professional content. More importantly, the book also showcases China's achievements in public health and its ongoing efforts within the Belt and Road Initiative, making significant contributions to the building

后　记

本书最初的创意始于 2021 年 9 月 27 日，当时正值中国刚刚获得世界卫生组织关于消除疟疾的认证，需要探讨如何将中国在消除疟疾方面的经验与非洲同行分享，以及如何共同构建人类卫生健康命运共同体。在此背景下，来自上海市科学技术协会、上海科学技术出版社、中国疾病预防控制中心寄生虫病预防控制所（国家热带病研究中心）等单位的五位专家在上海科学会堂举行了一次"头脑风暴"会议。会上五位专家达成共识：几家单位合作做一本科普书，既能作为在非洲开展的疟疾防控科普教育活动教材，又要能向非洲的疟疾防控工作者分享中国消除疟疾的经验。

会后，我们确立了一个简单却深远的目标：采用中英双语的形式做科普，将中国在疟疾防控领域多年积累的宝贵经验分享给更多国家和地区，帮助全球人民更好地理解和应对这一长期威胁人类健康的疾病。为此，我们组建了一个由疟疾专家、撰稿人、年轻画家和编辑等成员组成的多元化创作团队。经过多次线上和线下会议的讨论，我们最终决定采用中英双语对照、图文并茂的形式，向读者展示中国民众和专家如何积极参与疟疾预防、医疗卫生机构如何有效应对疟疾流行，以及地方政府如何协调和管理疟疾防控工作等专业内容。更为重要的是，这本书还能展现中国在公共卫生领域的成就、在"一带一路"倡议中所做的持续努力，以及为推动全球健康共同体的建设做出的重要贡献。

在经过三年多的不懈努力，历经多次修订、文字打磨、邀请外部专家审稿、反复审阅、三审三校、排版等流程后，本书终于要出版问世。我们期望这本书能为不同国家的普通民众提供易于理解的疟疾防控知识，帮助疟疾流行区的专业人员学习中国成功消除疟疾的经验，并为这些国家的政府官员提

of a global health community.

After more than three years of relentless effort, including multiple revisions, text refinement, inviting external experts for review, repeated proofreading, and three rounds of editing, layout design, this book is finally ready for publication. We hope this book can provide easy-to-understand knowledge about malaria control for general public in different countries, help professionals in malaria-endemic regions learn from China's successful experiences in malaria elimination, and offer government officials in these countries reference strategies for governance. The cases and approaches of malaria elimination in the book not only highlight the scientific nature of China's control strategies but also reflect the results of efficient governance through the concerted efforts of people and experts in malaria-endemic areas under government leadership. This can be considered an exemplary model.

During the compilation of this book, we received active responses and support from many malaria experts across the country. Particularly in the context of the global COVID-19 pandemic, the first five editorial meetings were conducted online. Despite geographical challenges, the core team maintained close communication, repeatedly discussing the details of illustration designs and planning schemes to present the best possible work.

On April 25, 2023, the book's album debuted at the "One River, One Belt, Together for a Malaria-Free World" special event in Shanghai. This event coincided with World Malaria Day and the tenth anniversary of the Belt and Road Initiative, giving it special significance.

The publication of this book was supported by National Key Research and Development Program (2023YFC2300800, 2023YFC2300804); the International Joint Laboratory on Tropical Diseases Control in Greater Mekong Subregion (No. 21410750200); National Key Laboratory of Intelligent Tracking and Forecasting for Infectious Diseases; Key Laboratory on Parasite and Vector Biology, Ministry of Health; WHO Collaborating Centre for Tropical Diseases and National Center for International Research on Tropical Diseases, Ministry of Science and Technology.

Here, we express our most heartfelt thanks to all participants and supporters!

Editorial Committee

供可借鉴的治理策略。书中所展示的消除疟疾案例和方法，不仅彰显了中国防控策略的科学性，也体现了疟疾流行区民众和专家在政府领导下齐心协力、高效治理的结果，堪称典范。

在本书的编纂过程中，我们得到了国内众多疟疾专家的热烈响应和支持。特别是在全球新冠疫情大流行的背景下，前五次编者讨论会都是通过线上方式进行的。尽管面临地域上的挑战，主创团队始终保持紧密的沟通，对插图设计和策划方案的细节反复讨论，力求呈现出最佳的效果。

2023 年 4 月 25 日，本书的同名画册在上海举办的"一江一河，一带一路，共创无疟世界"专题活动中首次公开展示，此次活动正值世界疟疾日和"一带一路"倡议十周年，具有特殊的意义。

本书的出版得到了国家重点研发计划（2023YFC2300800，2023YFC2300804）、上海市"科技创新行动计划""一带一路"国际合作项目"热带病防治澜湄联合实验室"（No.21410750200）、传染病溯源预警与智能决策全国重点实验室，国家卫生健康委员会寄生虫病原与媒介生物学重点实验室，世界卫生组织热带病合作中心，科技部国家级热带病国际研究中心等的资助。

在此，我们向所有参与者和支持者表示最衷心的感谢！

编委会

图书在版编目（CIP）数据

疟疾能在地球上消失吗？/ 周晓农主编 . —上海：上海科学技术文献出版社，2025

ISBN 978-7-5439-9039-5

Ⅰ . ①疟… Ⅱ . ①周… Ⅲ . ①疟疾—防治—中国 Ⅳ . ① R531.3

中国国家版本馆 CIP 数据核字（2024）第 086469 号

责任编辑：付婷婷
插　　画：张子扬
封面设计：颂煜文化

疟疾能在地球上消失吗？
NÜEJI NENGZAI DIQIU SHANG XIAOSHI MA
周晓农　主编
出版发行：上海科学技术文献出版社
地　　址：上海市淮海中路 1329 号 4 楼
邮政编码：200031
经　　销：全国新华书店
印　　刷：上海华业装璜印刷厂有限公司
开　　本：720mm×1000mm　1/16
印　　张：12.5
字　　数：158 000
版　　次：2025 年 3 月第 1 版　2025 年 3 月第 1 次印刷
书　　号：ISBN 978-7-5439-9039-5
定　　价：98.00 元

http://www.sstlp.com